End-of-Life Care and Addiction

A Family Systems Approach

Suzanne Young Bushfield, PhD, MSW, is a Licensed Clinical Social Worker who has worked with families for over 25 years in the fields of end-of-life care, health care, and mental health. She is a social work educator and researcher, and works as an Accreditation Specialist for the Council on Social Work Education. Suzanne has served on the faculties of the University of North Dakota, Lewis Clark State College in Idaho, Arizona State University, and New Mexico State University, and has participated in the CSWE–Gero-Ed Center initiatives funded by the John A. Hartford Foundation.

Brad DeFord, PhD, M Div, writes about aging, addiction, spiritual development, and end-of-life care. Through his private practice, Thresholds, he is a certified transitions consultant and life coach. He is also certified as a Level One Hospice Manager through The National Hospice and Palliative Care Organization (NHPCO). Brad has been a church pastor, a hospice chaplain, and the leader and developer of a bereavement program. For 6 years he served as the Leader of the Spiritual Caregiver Section of the National Council of Hospice and Palliative Professionals (NCHPP). Brad holds advanced degrees from Union Theological Seminary in New York and the Divinity School of the University of Chicago.

End-of-Life Care and Addiction

A Family Systems Approach

SUZANNE YOUNG BUSHFIELD, PhD, MSW
BRAD DeFORD, PhD, M Div

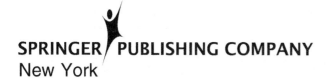

SPRINGER **PUBLISHING COMPANY**
New York

Throughout this volume various excerpts appear from *Opening Our Hearts, Transforming Our Losses*, copyright 2007, by Al-Anon Family Group Headquarters, Inc. Reprinted by permission of Al-Anon Family Group Headquarters, Inc. Permission to reprint these excerpts does not mean that Al-Anon Family Group Headquarters, Inc. has reviewed or approved the contents of this publication, or that Al-Anon Family Group Headquarters, Inc. necessarily agrees with the views expressed herein. Al-Anon is a program of recovery for families and friends of alcoholics—use of these excerpts in any non Al-Anon context does not imply endorsement or affiliation by Al-Anon.

Springer Publishing Company, LLC
11 West 42nd Street
New York, NY 10036
www.springerpub.com

Acquisitions Editor: Jennifer Perillo
Production Editor: Pamela Lankas
Cover design: David Levy
Composition: International Graphic Services

Ebook ISBN: 978-0-8261-2142-4

09 10 11 12/ 5 4 3 2 1

The author and the publisher of this Work have made every effort to use sources believed to be reliable to provide information that is accurate and compatible with the standards generally accepted at the time of publication. The author and publisher shall not be liable for any special, consequential, or exemplary damages resulting, in whole or in part, from the readers' use of, or reliance on, the information contained in this book. The publisher has no responsibility for the persistence or accuracy of URLs for external or third-party Internet Web sites referred to in this publication and does not guarantee that any content on such Web sites is, or will remain, accurate or appropriate.

Library of Congress Cataloging-in-Publication Data

Bushfield, Suzanne.
    End-of-life care and addiction : a family systems approach / Suzanne Bushfield, Brad DeFord.
        p. cm.
    Includes bibliographical references and index.
    ISBN 978-0-8261-2141-7 (alk. paper)
    1. Substance abuse—Social aspects. 2. Addiction—Social aspects. 3. Terminal care. 4. Families. I. DeFord, Brad. II. Title.
    HV4998.B87 2010
    362.17'5—dc22
                            2009036398

Printed in the United States of America by Hamilton Printing

I would like to dedicate this book to my own family, whose emotional process has made me who I am today.

—B. D.

I would like to dedicate this book to my husband, Bob; and my family who have always encouraged and supported me, and from whom I first learned what it means to be part of a family system.

—S. Y. B.

We also dedicate this book to those who work with families facing end-of-life and addiction.

—B. D. & S. Y. B.

Contents

Preface

This book began with a simple observation we repeatedly encountered in our work with hospice teams: Providing care to patients and their families was different somehow when those patients and/or families had histories of addiction. We noticed that certain discernable patterns were repeated, to the extent that when a family entered hospice care, someone on the team thought the new family was similar to another family we had served not long before. "This Jones family? They are an awful lot like the Smiths," would characterize the typical case presentation. And we would worry that we were not treating each family as its own discrete entity—but sure enough, soon the Joneses would indeed begin looking to us very much like the Smiths.

In our effort to understand what we were experiencing, certain discoveries emerged. For one thing, the medical model, common in hospice care, did not help us discover the uniqueness of each family. In part this is because the medical model is reductive: It only told us who the patient was according to the conclusions of his or her disease process. The medical model led us to have certain expectations of the persons who came onto our hospice services—mostly that they would die in a way appropriate to the course of the disease taking their life. There was, we supposed, a comfort in this—not for the person or the family, but for us, the members of the hospice team. Somehow being among so much death and dying was made more comfortable if, in some way, the processes we witnessed were predictable.

Unfortunately, that predictability led to disinterest. The end of some people's lives became "ho hum" for us because of the routine. However, when a disease took an unexpected turn, suddenly there were moments of interest again. We were interested because the way that particular person was dying was "different," and that difference caught our attention.

By the same token, one might think that the patients and/or families with histories of addiction would have sparked the interest of the hospice team. But the team's habit of categorizing them in terms of other, allegedly similar families diminished this interest. Instead, the team sought the comfort of familiarity and predictability. More surprisingly, a sense of blame or judgment often entered into our discussions about these families. We began to wonder why this was the case.

This wonder led us to the research and writing of this book. We began to organize our ideas, and to present them at clinical team conferences of the National Hospice and Palliative Care Organization. There, our ideas were well received. Workshop participants repeatedly told us that they needed to know more about providing end-of-life care to persons and families with histories of addiction. It is in no small part because of their encouragement that we are offering our ideas here.

One theme of this book is: "It takes two." First, we believe that it takes two *eyes* or points of view to see the patient and the family accurately. Our bodies are "stereoscopic": It takes two eyes to give us depth perception. In the same way, we say that it takes a stereoscopic vision to provide comprehensive end-of-life care.

On the one hand, we recognize that hospice care is a form and extension of medical care. It is for this reason that the medical model is used to direct patient care, and it is on the basis of a hospice's competence with the medical model that they are certified and accredited. Thus the medical model has its uncompromising importance in the delivery of end-of-life care. We affirm this.

On the other hand, the medical model itself is only one way to view the patient—and it almost never takes into account the family. We believe that end-of-life care is best practiced when both the patient and the family are taken into consideration. We advocate that the way to do this is to become knowledgeable about *families* and how they function. In this volume we offer family systems theory as one possible way to develop this understanding, but our point is more general. Taking families into account expands one's vision of the patient beyond whatever physical condition has brought him/her to the hospice service, and this provides a better, deeper, more human vision. This aim leads to the hospice maxim that the family is the "unit" or focus of care. It is our belief that this book will provide a better way for hospice teams to fulfill this goal.

We also explore a duality in the way information is presented here. In writing this book, we had much information to impart, but also had a story to tell. In fact, we had a number of stories, and we could not tell them all! So we decided to conflate our stories into one, and to complement our nonfictional information with the fictional account of one family—George, Wilma, John, and Amy Cinnamon. The Cinnamon family is *absolutely* fictional, but based on our observations of families treated in hospice. Likewise, we created a fictional hospice, which we call "Heart of Gold," staffed with fictional professionals. These characters are intended to play representative and illustrative roles (and are not intended to represent any persons living or dead) in our explanation of end-of-life care rather than reflect any specific individuals.

The theme of "it takes two" also relates to the *ears* we bring to end-of-life care, especially when it comes to listening to addicts and their families. We have the clinical ear that listens to our patients and families, and understands what they are saying. The other ear is the "ear" of the heart. This ear not only hears what they are saying and understands what they mean, but it also listens with compassion.

As we listened to patients and families with a history of addiction, we came to understand that what set them apart was the degree of *shame* they felt. The more we listened, the more we were convinced that providing compassionate end-of-life care meant responding in appropriately caring ways to this shame.

We learned that the Chinese character for "shame" (ch'ih) depicts a heart next to an ear (Whitehead & Whitehead, 1995, p. 90). We believe that it is through listening with the "ear" of the heart, hearing about and accepting another in the shame of their vulnerability with both humility and grace, that end-of-life care is best accomplished.

Further, "it takes two" applies very much to the collaboration that went into the writing of this text. One of us is a social worker, the other a spiritual caregiver. It has taken two professions to make this book, as well as two minds, and two hearts. We have experienced the benefits of dialogue. But we are not merely two people talking—we are two joined in the singular experience of life that is *conversation*.

Our conversations have been lively at times. We have different traditions, styles, and professional approaches, with overlapping theories, models, and approaches to people in their wholeness. Our commitment to holistic hospice care, to honoring the work of both recovery and dying, and to families whose stories live on beyond death, is what kept our conversation going. Here, we aim to share the fruit of that conversation, and to speak with one voice.

In offering this book, we are inviting others to join our conversation, too. Our obvious hope is not only to address those interested in end-of-life care and those concerned with addiction treatment and recovery, but also to bring people from those two fields of interest into conversation with each other. We believe that there is much we can learn from each other.

The most important thing of all we can learn from each other concerns the nature of family life. This book is for those who want to come to better understandings of their families—whether because there has been or is about to be a death in the family, or whether there is a history of addiction in the family, or simply because our families are worthy of our interest. What makes our families both interesting and our own is our family's story. We hope that what we offer here sparks sharing of families' stories and from that the discovery of how unique we are as well as how alike.

The final way in which this book "takes two" has to do with what is happening at this very moment. For it does take two—writer and reader—to make all of our stories come to life. We are grateful for your attention and hope that this volume offers you new ways to approach end-of-life care, addiction, and your families.

REFERENCE

Whitehead, J. D., & Whitehead, E. E. (1995). *Shadows of the heart: A spirituality of the negative emotions.* New York: Crossroads.

Acknowledgments

We would like to acknowledge those who have helped us along the way:

- The Betty Ford Center for the hospitality and pedagogy of its Professional In Residence program;
- The National Hospice and Palliative Care Organization for giving us the opportunity to present workshops at NHPCO conferences, where we initially shared many of the ideas that found their way into this book; the conversations were both helpful and encouraging;
- The courageous families we have had the privilege of knowing and serving:
  - ◆ families who have faced extraordinary challenges at the end-of-life, and in their grief;
  - ◆ families who have lived with addiction; and
  - ◆ families who have demonstrated enormous strength in recovery— living beyond grief, loss, and addiction; and
- The recovery community for its example and support.

End-of-Life Care and Addiction

A Family Systems Approach

1

Death and Addiction:
A Family Affair

George settled glumly into the passenger seat of the car, gathering the clear plastic tubing that ran from his portable oxygen tank to his nasal canula. His wife, Wilma, took her place behind the wheel, but made no attempt to drive. Neither spoke at first. They had just come from the oncologist's office, where the doctor had said, "George, I have run out of options for treating your lung cancer." George had asked, "Do you mean there's nothing more you can do for me?" The doctor had nodded her head, and said some other things, but he couldn't remember what they were.

Wilma did. She looked over at George and said, "I guess we better go home and call hospice, like the doctor suggested." She waited for George to respond. After what seemed like an eternity, George said, "I really could use a cigarette right now."

THE ROLE OF HOSPICE IN END-OF-LIFE CARE

The lives of George, Wilma, and their family have just taken a dramatic turn. George's oncologist had made a routine assessment by asking herself: *Would I be surprised if this patient died in the next 6 months?* Most likely, she admitted that she would not be surprised. This question

1

and its accompanying answer are what most often lead to a referral to hospice services.

What was a routine medical assessment for his oncologist, was an existential turning point for George. His life is now headed in a new direction, clearly toward its end. He and his entire family are going to be affected by this change in medical status.

Specifically, George's medical team will no longer try to *cure* George of his disease. Instead, they will concentrate on *caring* for him now that his prognosis is officially terminal. Once Wilma initiates hospice care for George, this shift will be underscored. *Caring* for people at the end of life is what hospice does best.

At the moment, George and Wilma are stunned and bewildered by this turn of events (even if, subconsciously, they had been anticipating it). Only gradually will the true meaning of this moment become apparent to them, and to the other members of their family. Hospice will help them discern that meaning and make the necessary life adjustments.

George and Wilma have become accustomed to the routines of medical treatment, as do most families in this situation. Their lives have been structured around doctor visits, hospital stays, and reactions to therapies. As fatiguing as it may have been, the rigors of seeking a cure gave George and Wilma, along with others in their family, something to do and talk about. Now, rather suddenly, much of that activity will stop, and what ensues is an unsettling stillness.

Their emotional and spiritual lives will also radically change. Up until now, George and Wilma have been hoping for (if not expecting) a cure and a return to their "normal" lives. Now that a cure will no longer be pursued, they are uncertain about what to expect and will need to begin adjusting their hopes.

Their lives are now fraught with unknowns, which can cause different fears and worries for everyone in the family. Fortunately, hospice professionals are familiar with a time in life that is unfamiliar to most. They are skilled at normalizing the end of life by providing information about what to expect.

Once George and Wilma invite a hospice team into their lives, they will initiate relationships that will last not only until George dies, but well into his survivors' mourning. When the Heart of Gold hospice team arrives, they will supplement the family's activities of care and support each member as he/she adjusts to this new, temporary way of living.

Accepting hospice care is not always easy. Initially, like many hospice users, George and Wilma may not be entirely clear about what a hospice team can do, nor what they *want* them to do. Moreover, because most hospice care occurs in the home, calling hospice means quite literally opening one's door to strangers. Families are expected to be welcoming and accommodating to hospice staff. Yet many feel that their privacy has been breached and their home invaded by hospice care.

Hospice professionals understand this. They understand that, in a symbolic way, an "invasion" has already occurred. For many families, hospice care represents not only the intrusion of death, but also its discomforting consequences. The arrival of the team and the materials they bring with them (new medications, medical equipment, a hospital bed) symbolize the disordering of people's lives brought about by a terminal prognosis, even as the team seeks to bring with it a sense that order can be restored.

The temporary relationships created by hospice care are extraordinary for all involved. As a result of hospice's interventions, the relationships among George and Wilma's family will be forever changed. Hospice care is an interactive experience of tremendous intimacy that often has life-altering consequences for the patient, the family, and even the hospice team. Hospice teams aim to accomplish this experience by focusing on the whole family. In hospice, there is a belief that "the family is the patient."

In our years of working with hospice teams, we have developed a deep appreciation for hospice. Given the complexities of end-of-life care, hospices do admirably well with the vast majority of the patients they serve, especially given the relatively brief time of that service. To function as well as they do, relationships and alliances need to develop quickly among the families, the patients, and the hospice team members. Hospice provides a crucible for caregiving relationships to begin, function meaningfully, and then end appropriately. Although most hospice teams do this exceedingly well, we believe that there is room for improvement.

Specifically, the shift in focus from the patient as an individual seeking a cure, to a family seeking care, is difficult to accomplish. There are reasons why many hospice teams tend to focus on *individuals* within the family system, instead of the system itself. One of the goals of this book is to shift the focus of attention to the whole system from that of its individual parts. If the family is truly to be the "unit of care," a grasp of "family systems" would therefore be essential not only to the care of George and Wilma, but also to all who enter hospice care.

To understand how and why hospices have difficulties regarding the family as the patient, we will begin this chapter by offering a brief history of hospice. We will then describe how hospice operates at the confluence of three fields: business, medicine, and psychosocial care. Psychosocial care in particular struggles to reconcile the competing interests of these fields (Healy, 2005; Taylor, 1998; Williams, 2003), as holistic approaches are more concerned with context and inherent values that may not be fully reflected in the other dominant and often competing fields (Healy, 2005).

Next, we discuss the application of family systems theory to hospice care, and how that approach can be particularly useful in families with histories of addiction. Understanding family systems is an essential tool for those engaged in end-of-life care, and even more so for families that have experienced addiction. We believe that a parallel process exists between hospice care and substance-abuse treatment. Similar to hospice services, substance-abuse treatment programs are medically based and medically guided businesses. In our opinion, however, recovery is not merely a matter of the efficacy of either business or medicine, but more a matter of the psychological and/or spiritual growth of the addict and the addict's family. Thus these concerns are common to both end-of-life care and addiction treatment.

Finally, we will discuss how a family systems approach may not only be useful in the care of hospice patients and their families, but also for understanding the functioning of the hospice team itself.

A BRIEF HISTORY OF HOSPICE

Although to date a definitive history of the hospice movement has not been written, what follows can suffice as a brief summary.

Hospice, as it is now practiced, has its roots in medieval times, when some monasteries set aside rooms for dying monks, and focused especially on their spiritual care. More recently, the contemporary hospice movement had its source in the pioneering work of Dame Cicely Saunders, a nurse and medical social worker who founded St. Christopher's Hospice in England in the 1960s. Saunders's effort to treat the dying with dignity by recognizing the limitations of medical interventions has had a lasting impact on end-of-life care throughout the world.

In the United States, recognition of her work roughly coincided with that of two other pioneers in changing dominant attitudes toward end of life. The impact of Elisabeth Kübler-Ross's *On Death and Dying* is well known. First published in 1969, Kübler-Ross's breakthrough was the affirmation of the humanity of the dying. She listened to people as they spoke about their feelings and experiences. She formulated what she called the "five stages" of dying: anger, denial, bargaining, depression, and acceptance. Kübler-Ross's research essentially founded an entire new field of study: *thanatology*, the study of death and dying, especially the psychological and sociological aspects of death.

Also among the notable early contributors to this field was Dr. Avery Weisman, a researcher at Massachusetts General Hospital, who spearheaded Project Omega. Project Omega studied the way cancer patients responded to their illness and its ramifications. Weisman's work led to what has come to be called *psycho-oncology*.

As the field of thanatology expanded, predominant cultural attitudes toward death and dying slowly started to change. What had begun as essentially a psychosocial–spiritual movement evolved further, as doctors and medical professionals became interested in thanatology. This gradually led to the establishment of hospices in the United States, many of which followed the model of St. Christopher's in England. Medical practices toward the terminally ill were examined and eventually altered, leading to the field of *palliative care*, a medical specialty that alleviates or manages pain. Even though the focus of palliative care extends beyond those who are dying to all who are in pain, it has in common with hospice the goal of *palliation*, which is the alleviation of suffering.

In 1982, the Medicare Hospice Benefit was enacted by Congress. This landmark legislation did two things: it established the four "core" hospice professional disciplines as medical, nursing, psychosocial, and spiritual care. It also provided criteria for reimbursement of hospice services, thus allowing hospices to become viable businesses.

HOSPICE AS A BLEND OF BUSINESS, MEDICINE, PSYCHOSOCIAL, AND SPIRITUAL SERVICES

Today, hospice, as it is practiced in the United States, blends the worlds of business, medicine, and spirituality. First, hospices are businesses. According to the National Hospice and Palliative Care Organization

(NHPCO, 2007), 92.6% of all hospice agencies were certified by the Centers for Medicaid and Medicare Services (CMS) to file for reimbursement under the Medicare Hospice Benefit, and 83.7% of hospice patients were covered by it. NHPCO estimates that in 2006, approximately 49% of hospices had not-for-profit status, whereas 46% were for-profit, and the remaining 5% were government-run programs such as those provided by the U.S. Department of Veterans Affairs. As an industry, hospice has grown to more than 4,500 programs since the first one was opened in 1974.

Most recent growth has been in small, freestanding programs. The median daily census in 2006 was 45.6 patients and only 16.2% of providers routinely [cared] for more than 100 patients per day (NHPCO, 2007). Industry growth is projected to be more likely in the for-profit sector than in nonprofits. Research indicates hospice's fiscal efficiency: "hospice services save money for Medicare" (NHPCO, 2007, p.5).

Most Medicare-certified hospices receive a per diem amount for each person receiving service, a rate of reimbursement determined annually by Medicare. Service must be provided for all patients and their families within that per diem multiplied by the average daily census over the course of the year. Some hospice patients' care costs more than others. A savings with one patient can be applied to the care of another, and differences are often offset by charitable donations.

Contracts are negotiated with providers outside the hospice, for example, with other businesses that provide durable medical equipment (DME) or oxygen or with pharmacies for commonly used medications. Sometimes, hospice teams discuss what changes might be made to the standard service "package" so as to remain competitive with other hospices in the area. Some medications are more expensive than others. For example, some hospices provide for ancillary needs (such as incontinence diapers and food supplements). Thus, although all hospices hold to certain standards, the range and quality of hospice services varies across hospices, just as it does in other businesses.

Costs per patient are monitored as long as patients are on service. Very short terms of stay are costly for hospices because initiating an admission is labor intensive. As patients remain on service, their costs may decline as their medical conditions are stabilized, or they may increase, if their medical conditions deteriorate. Costly patients who remain on service a long time deplete a hospice's assets. Less costly patients add to a hospice's bottom line and allow a hospice to manage and allocate its expenses better so as to meet the needs of other patients.

Second, hospices are medical care delivery systems. NHPCO estimates that 1.3 million patients received services from hospice in 2006, and that 36% of all deaths in the United States that year occurred under the care of a hospice program (NHPCO, 2007). The overall aim of contemporary hospice care is to provide the means for patients to die in the place they call "home." In 2006, nearly three quarters of all hospice patients died in a private residence, nursing home, or other residential facility, as opposed to an acute care setting (NHPCO, 2007). In contrast, in the general population about 50% of people die in acute hospitals. Almost 20% of all hospices operate a dedicated inpatient unit or facility; typically this inpatient care is provided by larger agencies with an average daily census greater than 200 patients (NHPCO, 2007). Less than 10% of hospice patients died in a hospital setting that was not managed by the hospice organization (NHPCO, 2007).

In the 1970s, when the hospice movement began in the United States, the majority of admissions were cancer patients. In the 1980s, a significant number of hospice admissions were patients with HIV/AIDS. Today, the hospice admissions profile has again changed. Only about one half of 1% of hospice patients are admitted with diagnoses of HIV/AIDS. And as deaths from cancer in the United States have declined to about 25% of all deaths, their proportion of the hospice census has declined as well. In 2006, about 44% of hospice patients were admitted with a cancer diagnosis. Significant among the noncancer diagnoses numbers were heart disease (12.2%); dementias, including Alzheimer's disease (10.0%); and lung disease (7.7%) (NHPCO, 2007).

Although hospice does offer service to younger persons (and has even established a field of pediatric hospice) over 80% of all hospice patients in 2006 were 65 and older, and about one third were over the age of 85 (NHPCO, 2007). This volume will focus specifically on hospice and end-of-life care for *older adult* patients and their families.

An analysis of Medicare beneficiaries over 65 who died in 2002 showed that females tended to use hospice more than males; Caucasians, more than people of color; and about 29% of older Americans made use of hospice for end-of-life care. More than other determining factors, hospice use was higher for "diseases that impose a high burden on caregivers, or diseases that predictably lead to death" (NHPCO, 2007, p. 7). The emotional and spiritual support that hospice offers to caregivers, along with their knowledge about the time frames of the courses of disease progression, are factors that attract families to hospice services.

Finally, hospice has a strong psychosocial and spiritual dimension, as demonstrated by the visionary work of Saunders, Kübler-Ross, Weisman, and others. As mentioned earlier, the Medicare Hospice Benefit affirms this dimension by including the provision of social work and spiritual care in hospice services.

NHPCO estimates that about three quarters of hospice employees provide patient care and/or bereavement support. According to NHPCO figures, nurses are the largest percentage of employees and physicians the smallest, with social workers falling in between. Chaplains and spiritual caregivers are regarded as essential by the Medicare Hospice Benefit, but this aspect of hospice care is not institutionalized in a uniform way. (For example, there are no NHPCO figures available for actual standard caseloads of chaplains, as there are for nurses, social workers, and home health aides. There are, however, "Guidelines for Spiritual Care in Hospice," which reflect Medicare Benefit guidelines for chaplaincy caseloads.) Across the spectrum of hospices, the relative emphasis on spiritual care, as well as on psychosocial services, varies greatly (Williams, Wright, Cobb, & Shields, 2004).

Still, NHPCO figures show that the bereavement services hospice provides average about two family members per death, and that "most agencies (93.9%) also offer community-wide bereavement programs" (NHPCO, 2007, p. 5). In addition, hospices benefit from the service of over 400,000 volunteers, who provide an estimated 5.1% of all clinical staff hours. The majority (58.9%) of volunteers assist in providing direct patient care, and the remainder provide general support (e.g., in fundraising or serving on hospice boards). Many, if not most, of these volunteers come to hospice to serve because they themselves and/or their families were served by hospice. Thus the number of hospice volunteers illustrates the efficacy of hospice in providing end-of-life care and its availability to provide continuing emotional and spiritual support to those who grieve.

THE HOSPICE TEAM AND MEDICAL, BUSINESS, PSYCHOSOCIAL, AND SPIRITUAL SERVICES

After Wilma called Heart of Gold Hospice, an admissions team of Susan (a nurse) and Bill (a social worker) were sent to their home. Together, they conducted the admission: Susan filled out the paperwork, reviewed George's medications, and interviewed both George and Wilma about his medical condition. Bill began to get to know them as people. He asked George what he wanted most at the moment—and George said, "A cigarette." Bill laughed, and said, "If I were going onto hospice, I'd start smoking again, too!" While he and Susan and George talked about how George's smoking could be managed, Wilma was distracted by other thoughts. George's smoking had long been a sore point. Now not only would he be smoking again, but they would have a noisy oxygen machine in their home! Wilma was not pleased with how things were going.

When they reported George's admission at the team meeting, Susan began with her assessment of his medical needs, including adjustments in his medications. She presented her nursing plan of care for review by the medical director and the other nurses on the team. Bill followed with his social work assessment of George, and his recommended plan of care.

The interplay of business, medical, and psychosocial issues can be seen in our fictional account of the Heart of Gold team meeting. First, the business realities of providing care are addressed at George's admission, and indeed they underlie every team discussion of every patient. Heart of Gold is a not-for-profit hospice, but it still needs to conduct itself in a fiscally responsible fashion.

Second, the language typically used to discuss persons and families on hospice service is primarily medical. For instance, Susan's presentation of George sets the tone for all other discussions, even those that are psychosocial-spiritual in content. George is the "patient"; Wilma is "family." As the patient, George receives the lion's share of attention during the team meeting. The medical aspects of his care will be the primary focus of the discussion whenever his case is reviewed and, sometimes, if there is no change in his medical status, the team will direct its attention to the next patient without pausing to ask the question, "How is the family doing?" In other words, the medical focus of hospice end-of-life care is on the patient as an individual and on the disease process in that patient's body.

It is our contention that, although business and medical issues are important to hospice care, and indeed necessary to their success as institutions, the discourse of the psychosocial and spiritual disciplines are most true to hospice's original intent and purpose. Yet, because the medical and business concerns often predominate in hospice practice, the psychosocial and spiritual disciplines are less likely to be heard.

For example, when George received a terminal prognosis, theoretically he stopped being a "patient" and could now be perceived again as a "person" who happened to be living out the end of his life. Moreover, as a person, he need not be singled out from his family (as he was, to a certain degree, when he was a patient) but could be restored to his family, once again a member of a greater whole. Indeed, this is how hospice would profess to regard him; for ideally in hospice, "the family is the patient." Unfortunately, neither the language of business nor the language of medicine facilitate George (and his family) being perceived in that way. Both treat George, in their own ways, as an individual: a patient in a business sense is a unit of reimbursement; a patient in a medical sense is a disease process or a diagnosis.

Too often, the voices of the business and medical perspectives drown out the psychosocial and spiritual voices central to hospice care. Yet, only the psychosocial and spiritual disciplines contain the language necessary for describing George as a person, and in the context of his family. Our question is: *Why is it that this happens so seldom?* Why is it that the psychosocial and spiritual disciplines often fail to articulate the perspective most original to hospice?

TOWARD A FAMILY SYSTEMS APPROACH TO END-OF-LIFE CARE

A psychosocial, spiritually focused hospice service would operate quite differently than what we fictionally described earlier in the chapter. In team meetings, for example, if George's status as a patient were secondary to the family's status as a group living through the imminent death of one member and the grief of the survivors, then the sequence with which these matters were discussed would be the opposite of what is typically practiced now.

On the other hand, our sense from working with hospice teams is that even when the psychosocial and spiritual matters are discussed, they are not as complete as they could be. As most commonly practiced, they, too, tend toward assessments based on individual psychology and personal spirituality. Thus, they still often lack a framework that enables them to speak of the family as a whole.

It is for these reasons that we are proposing family systems theory as a model for hospice end-of-life care, for all members of the hospice team. As originally conceived by Murray Bowen, family systems theory is a theory of human behavior that views the family as an emotional unit and uses systems thinking to describe the complex interactions (Kerr & Bowen, 1988) within that unit. To give just one example of how this shift in theoretical perspective can change a team's treatment of a family, we offer this: *From a family systems perspective, a death in a family is less an individual experience than an event experienced by everyone in the family.* Instead of focusing just on the individual and the changes in his or her body, mind, and spirit as he or she dies, a family systems approach recognizes how each member of the family responds to this imminent loss. This approach recognizes the emotional processes of the family prior to the diagnosis, and assesses the impact of this transition on all of the persons enduring it.

FAMILY SYSTEMS THEORY AND
FAMILIES WITH HISTORIES OF ADDICTION

This approach is especially needed, we believe, when offering care to families with histories of addiction. Whether the patient who comes to the hospice service is (or was) an addict, or whether there is another identified addict in the family, the addict tends to be somewhat isolated from the rest of the family. In our experience, this mimics the typical approach of substance-abuse treatment; addiction is spoken of as a disease of the family, but for the most part is treated as if it were the disease of the individual. The same is often true of hospice care.

We believe that end-of-life care and addiction treatment, seemingly two disparate fields, have much in common. Both would benefit from understanding that the *family is the patient*; the *family* is the unit of care. Both address aspects of human experience (dying, substance abuse) that carry with them a certain stigma.

When these two aspects of the human experience overlap—when the family with a history of addiction finds one of its members is dying—aspects of each are revealed that would become helpful to both, if they could learn from each other. We believe that a *family systems* approach to the end-of-life care for families with histories of addiction would significantly enhance both end-of-life care and addiction treatment.

In end-of-life care, for example, a family systems approach would allow the hospice team to speak of the family as a whole, and understand how addiction affects everyone in the family, not just the identified addict. This perspective is especially important because the hospice team's primary goal is not necessarily the "treatment" of the addicted individual but the guidance of the family through a major transition.

To return to our fictional example of George and Wilma, addiction has played a role in their lives that may not be readily apparent at first to the hospice team. As we (and the Heart of Gold hospice team) will eventually see, George has a history of alcoholism that has affected his family's dynamics for a long time; the implications of his addiction will continue to have an effect on how he and the family behave while he is on hospice. Originally, George's drinking brought him and Wilma together. Even though chemotherapy, radiation, and other treatments prompted him to curtail and later stop drinking ("I just don't have the stomach for it," George would say), the family patterns did not change. Thus Wilma's alcohol use might also be a concern for the hospice team. Our premise is that a family systems approach would help end-of-life professionals both identify and address aspects of addiction in a family's emotional process.

Why is it important to address histories of addiction in families under hospice care? Although no specific research has been done to identify the numbers of addicts and their families who have been served by hospice in any given year, it is more than likely that those numbers will increase. It is estimated that currently 1.7 million American adults over the age of 50 are substance dependent. This number is expected to increase to 4.4 million by 2020 (Farkas, 2008). If it is a reasonable assumption that addicts come to hospice care at rates approximately similar to the rest of the population, then hospice services can anticipate a parallel increase in the numbers of addicts they serve. It is also likely that a greater number of persons in recovery will require hospice service.

Substance-abuse treatment providers are already being advised to anticipate this increased need. One researcher describes what is to come as a " 'demographic tsunami' that requires additional attention to issues of substance abuse and commonly occurring medical disorders" (Bartels, 2006, cited by Farkas, 2008, p. 1) as our population ages.

At the same time, there is a concern that the substance-abuse treatment community will not recognize the magnitude of the issue. For one thing, most substance-abuse treatment centers tend to be aimed at younger persons. Concern has already arisen in social work circles for the adequate assessment of substance-abuse and dependency issues in gerontological populations (Axner, 2008). Unlike younger patients, older adult substance abusers are likely to display "lifetime patterns of drug use" and/or addictive behavior (Farkas, 2008). Second, substance abuse and chemical dependence in older populations tend to be "masked by other later life medical, social, and psychological problems" (Farkas, 2008, p. 1).

Additionally, prescription drug misuse and abuse may be mis- or underassessed, even more than alcohol abuse, illegal drugs, and other addictive behaviors. We have recently seen an increase in the availability and use of both "prescription and over-the-counter pharmaceuticals to treat illness and discomfort" (Farkas, 2008, p. 5). The likelihood that these medications will be misused or abused (intentionally or unintentionally) by older adults who come to hospice service is great.

The possibility of substance use or abuse has significant implications for all hospice professionals, which we will examine in more detail in later chapters.

FAMILY SYSTEMS THEORY AND THE HOSPICE TEAM

Finally, we believe that family systems theory benefits hospice teams not only in better understanding the people they serve, but also in better understanding *themselves*. Because hospice teams are their own systems, knowledge of family systems theory in particular, and an awareness of group dynamics in general, would help hospice teams improve their functioning.

Hospice teams are comprised of persons of diverse disciplines and backgrounds who are expected to function in such a way that the care they provide together is better than the care any of them could provide alone. They operate with an understanding that their specializations are complementary; that although their professional practices overlap to some degree, each is an expert in his or her own field.

Many hospice teams also commonly experience a sense of "family." For example, "family" is often the metaphor team members use to describe how they do (or should) relate to each other. A family systems perspective would help a hospice team better appreciate what being a "family" might mean. Once the team members have a sense of their own personal family's lives, they can gain a better understanding of what happens when their work "family" interacts with the families they serve on hospice.

Moreover, to some degree, in their work many hospice professionals bring to bear their own personal family experiences. This is of particular importance when hospice teams care for families with histories of addiction because many hospice professionals are themselves likely to be from families with histories of addiction (Baldisseri, 2007; Corsino, Morrow, & Wallace, 1996; Katsavdakis, Gabbard, & Athey, 2004; Smith & Seymour, 1985). In our experience, this correspondence may lead to *under*identification of the presence of addiction in families and, paradoxically, *over*reaction to some behaviors in those families. On the one hand, there may be such familiarity with the addictive family's dynamics that hospice professionals do not notice anything out of the ordinary. On the other hand, it becomes all the more important for hospice professionals to have a comprehensive understanding of their own experience so that they can treat others objectively.

A third dimension of this dynamic returns to how hospice professionals relate to one another as a team. All of us learn initially how to interact within a system from our families. Those whose families have histories of addiction have a different experience of what it *means* to be family than those who lack that history. Accordingly, the quality of teamwork depends on the family histories of those who come together to form a team.

CONTENTS OF THIS BOOK

The remaining chapters will elaborate on many of the concepts raised here. In chapter 2, we address appropriate adjustments in treatment (especially in medication adjustment) when there are histories of addiction in the patients (or the family members) who come under hospice care. In chapter 3, we discuss some physiological, psychological, and spiritual aspects of addiction. These chapters are by no means meant to be exhaustive. They are intended to provide a basic background within which addictive persons and their families might be better understood, especially by end-of-life professionals who may not be familiar with the dynamics of addiction and its treatment.

Chapters 4 to 7 of the book address key aspects of families, addiction, caregiving, grief, and loss. Certain typical emotional processes occur in all members of the family whenever one member receives a terminal prognosis. In chapter 4, we provide key characteristics of family emotional process that may help hospice better serve families at the end of life. We consider this same situation in families with histories of addiction in chapter 5. Because our premise is that families with histories of addiction react differently than families without such histories, we will explore how the emotional processes and dynamics differ. We will introduce the concept of *addiction emotional process* to describe this difference in family systems' terms. Also, we will show how the genogram can be used to depict these emotional processes.

With the admission to hospice, a partnership of caregiving begins. Providing caregiving to a dying family member presents its own challenges to the ones providing the care and to the one receiving the care. Hospice promises to expand the circle of care, beyond family and friends, to include the hospice team. As we will see in chapter 6, a systems approach appreciates what it takes to achieve this partnership.

The prospect of a death in the family creates a kind of a "clearing" within the emotional processes of that family. It offers an opportunity for things to be said that perhaps have gone unsaid; for emotions to be felt that perhaps have been suppressed or denied; and for relationships to be changed or rearranged. Many families experience an almost ominous quality during this period; as the finality of the situation becomes more apparent, a sense that this is their "last chance" arises. In families with histories of addiction, this moment amplifies dynamics that have distressed them throughout their history. The wounds of a history of abuse, neglect, or abandonment (which as we will see, are prevalent in such families) bring their own pain to what is often an already painful time. In chapter 7, we look at grief and mourning from a family systems perspective and see how it applies, in particular, to families with histories of addiction. We will show how using a systems approach might improve hospice's bereavement care with these families.

Next, we turn our attention to the hospice team. As stated earlier, many hospice teams also consider themselves a kind of "family." We will describe applying a systems approach to the functioning of hospice teams in chapter 8. In chapter 9, we examine how having a family with a history of addiction can have an impact on how team members work together.

As mentioned earlier, end-of-life care and addiction treatment share certain similarities; in particular, both carry with them a sense of taboo. Perhaps this is the reason that they are not usually addressed together, as we are doing here. Certainly, both the experiences of being addicted and of coming to the end of one's life bring with them a common experience of *shame*. In our society, there are often layers of shame that accompany a terminal prognosis, including a sense of shame over mortality as such. Matters of shame are woven throughout the fabric of addiction, its experience, and its treatment. In our final chapter we address this overlap.

Finally, in the Afterword, we review our interpretation of The 12 Steps and reflect on them in terms of how they might contribute to a deepened experience of the end of life. This book is intended not just for the members of families with histories of addiction, but for all persons—those dying, and those caring for the dying, whether as laypersons or professionals.

SUMMARY: WHAT FAMILIES WITH HISTORIES OF ADDICTION CAN TEACH US

In our willingness to address addiction and dying, we encourage others to speak candidly about their family histories and personal experiences with their health care providers, so that we might all give (and receive) better health care. This is especially important when it comes to end-of-life care. Health professionals who address this phase of care participate in an historic moment in a family's life. Our goal is to improve treatment and understanding and to provide adequate theoretical bases for addressing shame and abating judgment.

Our aim is to learn as much as we can about living, caring, and loving. Families with histories of addiction can teach us not only about themselves, but also about what it means to be a *family* in general. We believe that persons in recovery teach us not just about what it takes to recover from addiction, but also, perhaps, what it is to face one's own mortality, and thus to make the most of the last chapter of one's life. Of course, from everyone hospice serves, we learn what it means to participate in the human family.

REFERENCES

Axner, S. (2008). Substance use and abuse among older adults: Reflections from an MSW student. *Aging Times, 4*(2), 1–2.

Baldisseri, M. R. (2007). Impaired healthcare professional. *Critical Care Medicine, 35* (2), S106–S116.

Bartels, S. (2006). The aging tsunami and geriatric mental health and substance abuse. *Journal of Dual Diagnosis, 2*(3), 5.

Corsino, B., Morrow, D. H., & Wallace, C. H. (1996). Quality improvement and substance abuse: Rethinking impaired provider policies. *American Journal of Medical Quality, 11*(2), 94–99.

Farkas, K. (2008). Aging and substance use, misuse, and abuse. *Aging Times, 4*(2), 1–7.

Healy, K. (2005). *Social work theory in context.* New York: Palgrave MacMillan.

Kerr, M. E., & Bowen, M. (1988). *Family evaluation.* New York: W.W. Norton.

Katsavdakis, K. A., Gabbard, G. O., & Athey, G. I. (2004). Profiles of impaired health professionals. *Bulletin of the Menninger Clinic, 68*(1), 60–72.

Kübler-Ross, E. (1969). *On death and dying.* New York: Scribner.

National Hospice and Palliative Care Organization. (2007). *NHPCO facts and figures: Hospice care in America.* Washington, DC: Author.

Smith, D. E., & Seymour, R. (1985). A clinical approach to the impaired professional. *International Journal of Addictions, 20*(5), 713–722.

Taylor, S. (1998). A case of genetic discrimination: Social work advocacy within a new context. *Australian Social Work, 51*(1), 51–57.

Williams, M. L., Wright, M., Cobb, M., & Shields, C. (2004). A prospective study of the roles, responsibilities and stresses of chaplains working within a hospice. *Palliative Medicine, 18*(7), 638–645.

Williams, S. (2003). *Medicine and the body.* London: Sage.

2

Addiction Treatment: What Every End-of-Life Care Professional Should Know

Cigarettes were not the only thing George craved after he and Wilma left the oncologist's office. As soon as he got home, he poured himself a drink. Wilma started to object. "It's not happy hour," she said. George agreed: "No, it isn't a happy hour at all." Wilma quickly saw the truth in what George had said—and poured herself a drink, too.

In their initial meeting, Susan, RN, and Bill, SW, from the Heart of Gold hospice team had no way of understanding the role alcohol played in the lives of George and his family. This is not unusual because the significance of alcohol and drug use and abuse is often overlooked, denied, or simply not assessed by medical professionals (Center for Substance Abuse Treatment [CSAT], 2008).

Yet alcohol and drug use and abuse are increasingly prevalent among individuals and families, and it is important to assess and treat this behavior in end-of-life care. Because addiction often begins early in life, its presence in older adults has only recently received attention. In the material that follows, we focus primarily on addiction among older adults, because they are more likely to become hospice patients. Yet we also address addiction among other age groups because family members of hospice patients may also be experiencing effects of addictions.

In this chapter we provide some diagnostic criteria for recognizing and identifying addiction; address the impact of addiction among other family members; present the disease model of addiction, and compare it with other models; and examine best practices for assessing and treating addicted persons. Although an exhaustive discussion of addiction treatment is beyond the scope of this book, our goal is to provide sufficient information so that end-of-life professionals are better able to address the presence of addiction in the persons and families whom they serve through hospice care.

THE PREVALENCE OF ADDICTION AMONG OLDER ADULTS

Alcohol and prescription drug use are among the fastest growing health problems facing our country (SAMHSA, 2007). Aging does not deter nor abate alcohol and/or drug abuse. The pervasiveness of addiction among people age 60 and older in the United States is thought to be as high as 17% (SAMHSA, 2007). Prescription drug misuse and abuse is a growing problem among older adults in part because these drugs are more frequently prescribed for older adults, who are more vulnerable to the effects of drugs as they age (SAMHSA, 2007).

Many of the models for defining and classifying addiction are static, and do not take into account age-related physical and psychosocial changes. This makes it more challenging to identify addiction in older adults (CSAT, 2008). For example, anxiety and insomnia, two common diagnoses among older adults, are frequently treated with benzodiazepines; and pain, associated with arthritis and other age-related conditions, is frequently treated with narcotics. These are the same drugs most often linked to prescription drug addiction (Boston University School of Public Health, 2005).

Early use of alcohol is a very strong predictor of life-long alcoholism, although a third of all heavy drinkers begin their patterns of alcohol abuse after age 60 (Barrick & Connors, 2002). Addiction to prescription drugs, however, more typically begins later in life, when multiple losses arising from life changes can result in symptoms of depression. Due to some of the unique challenges faced by older adults (particularly isolation, changing body chemistry, more free time), it is expected that alcohol and drug addiction will increase 150% by 2020 (National Institute for Drug Abuse [NIDA], 2004). Yet currently, only about 3% of those seeking treatment for drug or alcohol abuse are over age 60 (Boston University School of Public Health, 2005).

Late-onset substance abuse is thought to be linked primarily to medical problems. Alcohol is the most commonly abused substance among the elderly, followed by painkillers and anti-anxiety drugs (Colleran & Jay, 2002). Blow and colleagues (Blow, Bartels, Brockman, & Van Citters, 2007) argue that "even as the number of (older) adults suffering from these disorders climbs, the situation remains underestimated, under-identified, under-diagnosed, and under-treated" (p. 1). It is disturbing that 20–25% of all patients with alcohol-related problems were treated medically for the symptoms of alcoholism rather than for the condition itself, and that a diagnosis of alcohol abuse was never made in almost one-fourth of all alcoholics seen for medical treatment (Backer & Walton-Moss, 2001). Other studies have more favorable results regarding assessment and accurate diagnosis, but primarily in younger persons with addiction. Although physicians are able to recognize substance abuse in approximately 60% of patients under the age of 60, they are accurate in recognizing substance abuse in only 37% of patients over the age of 60 (Meyer, 2005).

Why is addiction so easy to miss, especially among older addicts? A number of explanations have been offered. Sorocco and Ferrell (2006) suggest that there are two widely held myths regarding alcohol use: (a) that it is an infrequent problem and (b) that treatment success is limited. Physicians, trained in the more common and curable diseases, may therefore overlook addiction, particularly in older patients. Moreover, alcohol and drug abuse are still stigmatized by many. Therefore, some patients and their families may feel ashamed to discuss the problem with their physicians. By the same token, some health care professionals may be reluctant to raise the issue of substance use and abuse with their patients.

Those providing end-of-life care may be similar to the 81% of primary care physicians who do not regard themselves as prepared to identify alcoholism (NCASA, 2000). Perhaps underidentification is simply a matter that calls for better education. Whatever the reason, according to the National Center on Addiction and Substance Abuse (2000), 74% of patients who decided on treatment for their alcohol problems did so without the involvement of their primary care physician.

Hospice, although often associated primarily with cancer, treats people with a number of diseases. As discussed in chapter 1, about 44% of all hospice patients have a cancer diagnosis. Other common diagnoses include heart disease (12%), dementia (10%), and stroke (3.4%) (NHPCO, 2007). Cancer, heart disease, and stroke are known to be more prevalent among those who have addictions (Holman, 1996). Although these conditions have many contributing factors in addition to substance abuse, it does suggest that more people who have addictions will also present with the terminal illnesses that are common among hospice patients.

One area of increasing concern is the rise of opioid addiction. The prescription painkiller known as OxyContin is among the most abused prescription drugs; estimates are that 1.9 million people abuse it (CSAT, 2008). Because of its common use among hospice patients, issues regarding its control and administration have received attention. The FDA has strengthened its warnings about the drug (FDA, 2001) due to its abuse and diversion. Unfortunately, increased restrictions on its use may have a negative impact on hospice pain management. When used in terminally ill patients, opioid painkillers do not result in addiction (Manion, 1995; Sloan, Vanderveer, Snapp, Johnson, & Sloan, 1999; vonGunten, 2005), and hospice patients generally do not exhibit the drug-seeking behaviors common among nonhospice patients.

Nevertheless, many hospice patients have poor pain control, which is often attributed to their (or their caregivers') fear of addiction and tolerance (Tarzian & Hoffman, 2005; vonGunten, 2005). Recovering addicts, in particular, may fear or resist the use of pain medication (vonGunten, 2005). Increasingly, because of the rise of opioid misuse, hospice professionals may have concerns about other family members' and caregivers' use of drugs prescribed for the patient. For these reasons, hospice professionals should know how drugs are or have been used or abused in the past by *all* family members, not just the patient.

Although there is little statistical evidence of addiction among hospice patients, we believe that the "perfect storm" characterized by the predicted increase in addiction among older adults, the association of substance abuse with increased incidence of the diseases most commonly seen in hospice, and the demographic increase in older adults in general, make it increasingly likely that hospice professionals will encounter patients with some history of addiction. Even if hospice patients themselves do not present with histories of addiction, it is likely that members of their families will. Addiction issues can have an important impact on both the physical and psychological aspects of patients as well as their families at the end of life. Thus, hospice and palliative care personnel, along with other health professionals, would benefit from becoming more familiar with addiction identification and treatment.

Fortunately, through recent education programs and outreach efforts, health care professionals have received information about addiction screening and brief intervention. This information integrates problem and diagnostic approaches, using both the research literature and clinical experience to refine the methods of screening, referring, and treating persons with substance abuse (SBIRT, 2007). Health professionals who provide end-of-life care would benefit from this information. We hope this chapter will provide a basic introduction to this field.

THE DIFFICULTIES IN DIAGNOSING ADDICTION IN OLDER ADULTS

The *Diagnostic and Statistical Manual of Mental Disorders* (DSM IV-TR; APA, 2000) uses the following diagnostic markers to determine whether substance use or misuse is abusive: A maladaptive pattern of substance use leading to clinically significant impairment or distress by one or more of the following, occurring within a 12-month period:

1. recurrent substance use resulting in a failure to fulfill major role obligations at work, school, or home;
2. recurrent substance use in situations in which it is physically hazardous, such as driving or operating a machine while impaired;
3. recurrent substance-related legal problems, such as arrests for disorderly conduct; and
4. continued substance use despite having persistent or recurrent social or interpersonal problems caused or exacerbated by the effects of the substance, such as arguments with spouse about consequences of intoxication, or physical fights (APA, 2000, p. 199).

This last criterion can be summarized by an acronym often used by addiction professionals—CUDAC: *Continued use despite adverse consequences.* This is a hallmark of substance abuse, and one that often perplexes those who study addiction. Why do addicts persist, even in the face of increasingly dire consequences?

For the hospice professional, CUDAC may be excused in the context of death—why bother to address addiction when death is imminent? Yet even at this last stage of life, substance abuse may play a powerful and negative role in the life of the addicted person and his family.

Other signs of substance abuse may include: "slurred speech, lack of coordination, unsteady gait, memory loss, fatigue and depression, feelings of euphoria, and lack of social inhibitions" (APA, 2000, p. 197). Unfortunately, many co-existing age-related chronic conditions may mimic or mask signs of substance abuse, making diagnosis more difficult. For example, many older patients may experience diminished mobility and pain caused by arthritis, osteoporosis, and other skeletal system changes (Whitbourne, 2002). These may lead to unsteady gait. Declines in strength and endurance, which may lead to fatigue, deteriorating reflexes, and incontinence could reflect a change in the muscular system due to aging, not substance abuse (Whitbourne, 2002). Vision and hearing changes may contribute to balance problems and falls (Aldwin & Gilmer, 2004). Neurological injury or disease may lead to brain deficits which affect speech, memory, and mood (Whitbourne, 2002). Many of these age-related changes are exacerbated by lifestyle variables, which include addiction and substance abuse (Valliant, 2003).

Identification of addiction also relies on information from other sources: The addict may have work and family-related problems, or get arrested for driving under the influence. For older adults who are not working, are living alone, and are perhaps no longer driving—their addiction may remain hidden for longer periods of time (Colleran & Jay, 2002). Corroboration is a key aspect of diagnosis; significant others may provide collateral information which helps substantiate and authenticate other sources of information (Miller & Rollnick, 2002).

Often, the diagnosis of substance abuse is made following the identification of common comorbid disorders. However, this too is problematic among older adults. For example, malnutrition, which sometimes occurs in cases of substance abuse, may also occur in older adults with more frequency as a result of poverty, cognitive dysfunction, limited mobility (which restricts access to grocery shopping or ability to prepare meals) and problems with teeth or dentures. Poor nutrition may also come from other life changes and losses, such as when a spouse dies, and may be associated with depression (SAMHSA, 2007).

Accurate diagnosis of substance abuse is multifaceted: It includes an evaluation of history, signs and symptoms, laboratory and other diagnostic tests (Jacobson, 1983). A variety of screening tools attempt to provide valid, reliable, and practical measures to support the diagnosis. Laboratory tests include urine, blood, hair, saliva, and sweat tests, with varying abilities to detect positive levels of substances. However, such tests are used infrequently with older adults. The amount or frequency of substance use, metabolic rate, body mass, age, overall health, drug tolerance, and urine pH can all affect the detection periods and reliability of various lab measures. Ageist assumptions and attitudes may inhibit the use of such tests with older adults (Finlayson, 1998).

There are also cultural variations in attitudes toward substance use, patterns of use, reaction and prevalence of substance use. Thus evaluation of substance use "should always consider aspects of culture, gender, and age" (APA, 2000). Cultures differ in their values and communication styles, family structure, and in the role of alcohol and other substances in traditions, rituals, and family life. There are also cultural differences regarding aging itself. Some cultural groups hold elders in high respect (Huber, Nelson, Netting, & Borders, 2008), whereas many older adults in Western cultures experience a sense of being devalued. Further, substance abuse is disproportionately represented among some cultures. For example, Native Americans are six times more likely to die of alcohol-related causes than the general U.S. population (Frank, Moore, & Ames, 2000). Substance misuse has been tied to a sense of powerlessness and low self-esteem, which are also present among minority groups who experience cultural identity conflicts, discrimination, poverty, and stressors related to acculturation (Sue & Sue, 2008). Assessment and identification of substance abuse among ethnic elders may be challenging because of barriers in communication, cultural norms, and beliefs about the use of substances.

RECOGNIZING ADDICTION ISSUES IN FAMILY MEMBERS

Hospice professionals should be aware that addiction may be present in the patient, other family members, or caregivers. (We will elaborate on the impact of addiction on other family members in chapter 3). Addiction, when present in any member of the family, serves to complicate best practices both in hospice and addiction care. Patterns of substance abuse and addiction may be generational, which has its own impact on the family members' ability to identify problems with addiction objectively. And when older adults depend on family members for their care, it may be more difficult for them to do anything that jeopardizes their reliance on others, whether out of fear of retribution, protection, or rationalization (Miller & Rollnick, 2002). Families may have adapted to the addiction in a family member—exhibiting denial and making corroboration more difficult (Miller & Rollnick, 2008).

In our fictional example of George and Wilma, the Heart of Gold Hospice Team members did not initially realize that George meets the *DSM-IV* criteria for addiction and they might have missed Wilma's reliance on alcohol as well. However, they will learn that George and Wilma's son, John, definitely meets the *DSM-IV* criteria. Eventually, as the team comes to know the family better, they will recognize the importance of alcohol in the life of the entire family.

MODELS OF ADDICTION TREATMENT

The field of addiction treatment has been largely guided by three models: the moral model, the behavioral model, and the disease model. These conflicting models lead to very different approaches in the identification, treatment, and management of addiction.

Historically, *moral models* viewed addiction as a consequence of personal or character weaknesses, resulting from poor individual choices and a failure of will. Treatment was based on an understanding of addiction as a crime or a sin. The social aspect of the moral model included the need for religious interventions as well as a turning away from willful misconduct and/or the violation of societal norms.

In contrast, *behavioral models* treat addiction as a habit that is developed over time, and embedded in certain cultural frames, one that may have elements of both basic conditioning processes and social learning. In these models, education, retraining, development of new coping skills, willpower, and repair of relationships can be viewed as primary evidence of recovery. In this approach, cognitive processes can be restructured to counter the previously held thoughts linked to addictive behavior.

The model gaining ascendency in addiction treatment is the *disease model*. Disease models suggest that biological or neurochemical processes are the primary cause of addiction—not just the result. Research into genetics further suggests that there are inherent predispositions toward the disease of addiction, requiring management of risk factors and perhaps genetic counseling. This medical view of addiction focuses on the process of the disease of chemical dependency as essentially irreversible. Specific treatments or interventions, such as identification, detoxification, management of biomedical or behavioral complications, and even recovery, are built on the premise that the disease abnormality is primarily responsible for addiction. Many contemporary treatment services are based on the medical model of addiction.

We will discuss the disease model in more depth in chapter 3, and use it as the basis for our approach to end-of-life care and addiction throughout this book. We will often compare the contrasting (and sometimes competing) characteristics of the disease model and the family systems model (introduced in chapter 1). In chapters 4 and 5, we will propose the development of a broader understanding of addiction within a systems framework. We believe that treating addiction as an individual disease limits our understanding of addictions' systemic and family implications.

The three models yield very different attitudes toward addicts and addiction. For example, addicts may be treated with disdain by those who believe in the moral model, which likely only adds to the shame the addict already feels. The phenomenon of shame and addiction will be addressed from a system's perspective in chapter 5.

In the medical or disease-based model, the addict is treated as a person who is "sick" and seeking a "cure." The result is a confusing mixed message for addicts: On the one hand, the disease makes one a patient, meaning that the disease is the focus of treatment; to a degree this attitude is "de-personalizing." On the other hand, recovery encourages one to be a person, and to take responsibility for one's own behavior. This mixed message may also contribute to ambivalence about recovery and the recovery process on the part of the addict and the addict's family.

Likewise, a behavioral model suggests that the addict has chosen a particular behavior (i.e., substance abuse) and that by manipulating the addict, "control" of that behavior is obtained by those outside of the addict. The message implied is not one of empowerment. The behavioral model heightens individual responsibility, but apart from its social context. Thus the behavioral model can collapse into the moral model, for example, by insinuating that relapse is a failure of will. The behavioral model suffers from its lack of regard both of underlying causes and of overriding contexts.

As with all of us, people who struggle with addiction are embedded in social networks. These networks may have constructive or destructive influences upon them and their quests for health (Miller & Rollnick, 2002). In this text we are specifically interested in the influence on the addict of the social network of the family, which will be addressed in chapters 4 through 7.

BEST PRACTICES WITH ADDICTION: ASSESSMENT AND INTERVENTION IN THE HOSPICE SETTING

Assessing the use of alcohol and/or drugs is an essential first step to treating addiction. Measures of alcohol consumption may be used, including diaries, self-monitoring logs, and other self-report instruments. Structured clinical interviews that provide severity scores may also be useful. Common brief screening tools can be used or modified to screen for other drug use. These screening tools are based on asking specific questions, as the commonly used CAGE tool shows:

C: Have you ever felt you should Cut down on your drinking?

A: Have people Annoyed you by criticizing your drinking?

G: Have you ever felt bad or Guilty about your drinking?

E: Have you ever had a drink first thing in the morning to steady your nerves or get rid of a hangover (Eye-opener) (Hinkin et al., 2001; Jarvik, 2001; Mayfield, McCloud, & Hall, 1974, p. 1121).

However, there are some inherent problems with this tool's use with older adults who, due to isolation, may not experience the same social sanctions associated with addiction in younger populations.

The Michigan Alcohol Screening Test–Geriatric (MAST-G) version (Blow et al., 1992) is a widely used 24-item self-administered questionnaire. More complex than CAGE, it can also be used to guide a structured interview. The MAST-G is designed to determine common signs and symptoms of problem drinking and alcoholism, and the questions can also be modified to address drug use. This more detailed tool addresses issues pertinent to older adults. Examples from the MAST-G include: "Did you find your drinking (drug use) increased after someone close to you died?" and "When you feel lonely, does having a drink help?" (Blow et al., 1992). Other variations of these tools have also been developed to address special populations, such as women and adolescents.

Blood and urine tests may also be helpful in determining specific biological markers, but aging produces physical changes that lead to a lower tolerance for some substances (CSAT, 2008). Therefore, careful interpretation of laboratory results is needed.

Once identification of addiction is made through screening or other direct questions, hospice professionals can establish a relationship that will result in appropriate treatment and intervention for both the addict and the addict's family—even within the brief span of time associated with hospice care.

Significant therapeutic relationships often require an investment of time. However, the typical hospice patient receives services for only 20 days (NHPCO, 2007). This short time period suggests that hospice professionals need to be skilled in engagement and assessment, and be ready to intervene appropriately. Given the nature of end-of-life care, hospice professionals may wonder whether intervention can be both appropriate and effective. The data suggests that making appropriate responses can have a significant effect, even if the interval for action is brief.

For instance, brief interventions have been shown to be effective in reducing alcohol consumption, binge drinking, and the frequency of excessive drinking in problem drinkers (Fleming, Barry, Manwell, Johnson, & London, 1997). In fact, "even a one-time brief encounter of 15 minutes or less has been shown to reduce nondependent problem drinking by more than 20%" (SAMHSA, 2007, p. 454). Among older adults, two or three 10 to 15 minute counseling sessions are often as effective as more extensive interventions (Bien, Miller, & Tonigan, 1993).

This evidence would suggest, therefore, that intervention with addiction is not futile. However, different intervention approaches and perspectives may yield different results, and it is not known if results would vary within the context of end-of-life care. Completion rates using brief interventions are better for elder-specific alcohol programs than for mixed-age programs (Atkinson, 1995), and late-onset alcoholics are more likely to complete treatment and have somewhat better outcomes using brief interventions (Liberto & Oslin, 1995). Certainly, adaptation of existing models may be necessary to address the particular issues for addiction when co-occurring with families facing end of life.

SUGGESTED TREATMENT APPROACHES FOR END-OF-LIFE ADDICTION

Three strategies have been identified and supported by varying levels of research evidence, as effective interventions with addiction: motivational interviewing; cognitive-behavioral intervention; and "life-context" or person-in-environment approaches. In this section we will illustrate the ways in which these three different approaches can be translated into end-of-life care.

Motivational Interviewing

SAMHSA (2007) has developed, through a consensus panel of experts, treatment improvement protocols (TIPS) for substance abuse with older adults. One effective and recommended approach in addiction treatment is *motivational interviewing*. Motivational interviewing recognizes that a democratic partnership between the clinician and the addict can establish an environment that is empathic, supportive, and yet directive; it is thus more successful in achieving change (Miller & Rollnick, 1991, 2002). Described as "a way of being with a client" as opposed to a set of techniques, motivational interviewing emphasizes the *therapeutic* nature of the relationship. The sessions in this approach include a variety of foci, including motivation-for-change strategies, education, assessment of the severity of the problem, providing direct feedback, contracting and goal setting, behavioral modification techniques, and the use of written materials such as self-help manuals.

In describing the motivational interview, Connors, Walitzer, and Dermen (2002) indicate that it consists of the following:

1. eliciting self-motivational statements;
2. reflective, empathic listening;
3. inquiring about the client's feelings, ideas, concerns, and plans;
4. affirming the client in a way that acknowledges the client's serious consideration of and steps toward change;
5. deflecting resistance in a manner that takes into account the link between therapist behavior and client resistance;
6. reframing client statements as appropriate; and
7. summarizing (p. 1164).

The strength of motivational interviewing is that it addresses the human ambivalence toward change—even when the desire to change has been expressed. By viewing resistance as an equal-but-opposite force to the desire to change, motivational interviewing helps the clinician to build a relationship that expresses confidence in the individual's capacity to change for the better, thus enhancing their commitment to change. This intentionally supportive relationship can be effective even in the short term, and seems quite consistent with approaches generally used in hospice psychosocial care. Hospice professionals incorporate supportive counseling in their approaches to patients and families facing the difficult transitions related to death, dying, and bereavement. Their existing skills, therefore, may be transferable to skills in motivational interviewing directed at issues related to substance abuse.

Cognitive-Behavioral Therapies

Another approach is *cognitive-behavioral and self-management interventions* (CB/SM). Currently, CB/SM forms the basis of many treatment programs focused on substance abuse. Treatment from this perspective consists of four phases:

- Analysis of previous substance abuse behavior;
- Identification of high-risk situations (antecedents, behaviors, and consequences) of substance use;
- Skills training, to enhance coping with high-risk situations and relapse prevention; and
- Continuing care and follow-up (SAMHSA, 2007).

According to the CB/SM approach, the burden for behavioral modification is on the individual and the emphasis is on being accountable to oneself. In making the effort to change or alter behaviors that are objectively CUDAC (continued use despite adverse consequences), an individual is taught self-management techniques, such as how to recognize triggers for their substance use behavior, and how to remove themselves from those situations or use coping skills to address those stressors. The addict is encouraged to implement these strategies and is provided with supportive reinforcement for using them. The strength of the CB/SM approach is in promoting the individual's responsibility for oneself, and the evidence of its effectiveness is based on observation of objective changes in the individual's behavior.

Many CB/SM-based treatment programs recognize the emotional and familial aspects of addiction and addiction's consequent behaviors. For example, adult addicts in particular may have many issues related to multiple losses—having lost family members, social relationships, their health and social status, and their sense of self-worth. (We will discuss the relationship of addiction to loss more fully in chapter 5.) Clearly, one consequence of addiction includes impairment in significant relationships, including the alienation from family and friends. Many older adults have increased needs for medications (due to other health conditions associated with aging) which may complicate their relationship with drugs. Recognizing these factors takes into account the multifaceted nature of addiction and its consequences. Although most CB/SM-based addiction treatment programs focus primarily on the individual, they include both medical treatment and opportunities to interact in a small group setting. In these small groups, recovering addicts are taught social skills and mutual support. Family involvement tends to be used to inform the treatment counselor about the addict's history or to reinforce the behavioral approaches; but treatment is usually not directed at the family itself.

End-of-life professionals are familiar with educating patients and families about their health conditions, and helping them take control of self-management for their pain and other symptoms. They also commonly incorporate group approaches, psychoeducational support, and pay keen attention to how the patient and family are responding to changes associated with terminal illness and impending death. For all of these reasons, the skills and activities required by CB/SM approaches may already be familiar to many end-of-life professionals.

Life Context or Person-in-Environment Approaches

In contrast to motivational interviewing and CB/SM, there is some evidence that a person's relationship to others and to his environment can have significant influence on his behavior and his ability to change— even to recover from addiction. For example, Waldorf, Reinarman, and Murphy (1991) found that many addicted people with jobs, strong family ties, and other close emotional supports were able to end their addiction to cocaine. Addicts with stable lives, good jobs, supportive families and friends, college educations, and other social supports have a great deal to lose if they continue their substance abuse, and that may provide motivation to alter their drug-using behaviors (Cloud & Granfield, 2001).

It is unknown how one's impending death, or the death of a loved one, may alter the influence of other supportive aspects, because this topic has not benefited from research. But we anticipate that these same supports may have an impact on addiction, even as end-of-life concerns become important—or perhaps, *especially* as end-of-life concerns increase in importance

Social support, long recognized as essential to many coping strategies, is a concept that derives its meaning from competing philosophies. These competing philosophies focus more on the individual (and the individual's transactions with aspects of support) on the one hand, but also focus on larger systems (such as the family or community) and their influence on the individual, on the other hand. The *person-in-environment model* (Richmond, 1917) suggests that, instead of being mutually exclusive, there is an *interdependence* of both the person and the environment, thus a necessary interaction of each with the other.

The reciprocal impact of substance-abuse behaviors is supremely evident in family interaction patterns, and we will elaborate upon these interactions later in this volume. For the moment it is important simply to note that persons with addictions benefit from social support in order to maintain recovery, and at the same time they often have gaps in this very much needed support which, in turn, influences addictive behaviors.

At the very least, the person-in-environment model suggests that the interaction between a person with addiction and the family results in changes to *both* the person and the family, particularly through its patterns of relationship and communication. For the addict, there is both a greater need for support, and a greater likelihood that this support may be impaired by the effects of addiction. When this reality intersects with end of life, and its accompanying need for additional care and support, additional tensions are created. More evidence is needed to support the effectiveness of this model's success in addiction treatment. However, we suggest the following application of this principle to substance abuse and end-of-life care:

■ More attention to substance abuse in the elderly is needed by health and social service professionals and those who have contact with older adults, including hospice care providers.

■ Functional impairment, cognitive or memory problems, sleep disorders, and depression may have a relationship to substance abuse in the older adult. These symptoms warrant attention, particularly from hospice professionals who regularly assess these aspects of patient care. In addition, these should also be assessed as part of their care of family members and caregivers.

■ Hospice providers recognize that death and dying and the accompanying involvement of others can be overwhelming to the patient, and are skilled at making assessments of when the presence of others is or is not helpful to the patient's well-being. Involvement of only one or two relatives in intervention strategies may be more appropriate for older adults.

■ Age-specific interventions that are flexible, supportive, and non-confrontational are most effective with addiction; patient and family centered care from hospice professionals similarly is designed to support the individual's needs and wishes.

■ Focus on rebuilding the support network, identifying linkages with community-based, culturally relevant services and supports. This aspect of best practices in addiction with older adults coincides with the psychosocial care that extends, in hospice, beyond the death of the individual patient to the family in bereavement. Hospice professionals may therefore be well suited to adapt their understanding of bereavement care to the requirements for recovery from addiction.

SUMMARY: ADDICTION TREATMENT
AND END-OF-LIFE CARE

End-of-life care and addiction treatment share a sense of urgency brought on by the formidable prospect of change. When any us of are faced with change, our initial response is likely to be ambivalence. Because "it is when people get *stuck* in ambivalence that problems can persist and intensify," that "ambivalence can be a key issue that must be resolved for change to occur" (Miller & Rollnick, 2002, p. 14). Whether change is self-initiated (as it is frequently in recovery from addiction) or is prompted from external forces (as when one is given a terminal prognosis), how one responds to the prospect of change is the crossroads where addiction treatment and end-of-life care meet. To paraphrase what is usually said of fame: Some people choose change; others have change thrust upon them.

Because of this intersection, it is important to address how people react and respond to change. For hospice professionals, understanding how addicts and their families operate can be useful in understanding how families in general respond to change. In future chapters, we will examine why change of any sort, be it recovery or terminality, can be problematic for families.

When people come to the end of life, there tends to be an acceptance of existing ways of being: "Why bother to intervene, when someone has only a short time to live?" seems to be the question end of-life-care professionals tacitly ask. This reluctance to identify or intervene can be harmful in cases of addiction, just as it is also a missed opportunity in end-of-life care. Both addiction and end of life present opportunities for growth and transformation.

REFERENCES

Aldwin, C., & Gilmer, D. (2004). *Health, illness, and optimal aging: Biological and psychosocial perspectives.* Thousand Oaks, CA: Sage.

American Psychological Association. (2000). *Diagnostic and statistical manual of mental disorders* (4th ed., text rev., p. 197). Washington, DC: American Psychiatric Press.

Atkinson, R. (1995). Treatment programs for aging alcoholics. In T. Beresford & E. Gomberg (Eds.), *Alcohol and aging* (pp. 186–210). New York: Oxford University Press.

Backer, K. L., & Walton-Moss, B. (2001). Detecting and addressing alcohol abuse in women. *Nurse Practitioner, 26*(10), 13–22.

Barrick, C., & Connors, G. (2002). Relapse prevention and maintaining abstinence in older adults with alcohol abuse disorders. *Drugs & Aging, 19*(8), 583–594.

Bien, T. J., Miller, W. R., & Tonigan, J. S. (1993). Brief interventions for alcohol problems: A review. *Addictions, 88*(3), 315–335.

Blow, F., Brower, K., Schulenberg, J., Demo-Dananberg, L., Young, J., & Beresford, T. (1992). The Michigan Alcohol Screening Test–Geriatric version: A new, elderly specific screening instrument. *Clinical and Experimental Research, 16,* 372.

Blow, F., Bartels, S., Brockman, L., & Van Citters, A. (2007). *Evidence based practices for preventing substance abuse and mental health problems in older adults.* Center for Substance Abuse Treatment. Retrieved October 10, 2008, from http://www.samha. gov/Older AdultsTAC

Boston University School of Public Health. (2005, Nov.–Dec.). Elders with substance abuse. *Alcohol, Drugs and Health.* p. 1.

Center for Substance Abuse Treatment. (2008). *Substance abuse: Older adults at serious risk.* Retrieved October 3, 2008, from http://www.fda.gov/Safety/MedWatch

Cloud, W., & Granfield, R. (2001). Natural recovery from substance abuse dependency: Lessons for treatment providers. *Journal of Social Work Practice in the Addictions, 1*(1), 83–104.

Colleran, C., & Jay, D. (2002). *Aging and addiction: Helping older adults overcome alcohol or medication dependence.* Center City, MN: Hazelden.

Connors, G., Walitzer, K., & Dermen, K. (2002). Preparing clients for alcoholism treatment: Effects on treatment participation and outcomes. *Journal of Consulting and Clinical Psychology, 70*(5), 1161–1169.

Finlayson, R. (1998). Prescription drug dependence in the elderly: The clinical pathway to recovery. *Journal of Mental Health and Aging, 4*(2), 233–249.

Fleming, M. E., Barry, K .L., Manwell, L. B., Johnson, K., & London, R. (1997). Brief physician advice for problem alcohol drinkers: A randomized controlled trial in community-based primary care practices. *Journal of the American Medical Association, 277*(13), 1039–1045.

Frank, J., Moore, R., & Ames, G. (2000). Historical and cultural roots of drinking problems among American Indians. *American Journal of Public Health, 90*(3), 344–351.

Hinkin, C., Castellon, S., Dickson-Fuhrman, E., Daum, G., Jaffe, J., & Jarvik, L. (2001). Screening for drug and alcohol abuse among older adults using a modified version of the CAGE. *American Journal on Addictions, 10*(4), 319–326.

Holman, R. (1996). Zenaca logs higher sales. *Wall Street Journal, 228*(86), 18.

Huber, R., Nelson, H. W., Netting, F. E., & Borders, K. (2008). *Elder advocacy: Essential knowledge & skills across settings.* Belmont, CA: Brooks Cole.

Jacobson, S. W., Jacobson, J. L., & Sokol, R. J. (1983). *Substance abuse and parenting.* Washington, DC: Alcohol, Drug Abuse and Mental Health Administration.

Liberto, J., & Oslin, D. (1995). Early versus late onset of alcoholism in the elderly. *International Journal of the Addictions, 30*(13-14), 1799–1818.

Manion, J. C. (1995). Cancer pain management in the hospice setting. *Minnesota Medicine, 78*(2), 25–28.

Mayfield, D., McCloud, G., & Hall, P. (1974). The CAGE questionnaire: Validation of a new alcohol screening instrument. *American Journal of Psychiatry, 131,* 1121–1123.

Miller, W. R., & Rollnick, S. (2002). *Motivational interviewing* (2nd ed.). New York: Guilford Press.

Miller, W. R., & Rollnick, S. (2008). *Motivational interviewing* (3rd ed.). New York: Guilford Press.

National Center on Addiction and Substance Abuse. (2000, April). The economic value of excessive drinking. *National Center on Addiction and Substance Abuse Newsletter.* New York: Columbia University, April, 2004.

National Hospice and Palliative Care Organization. (2007). *NHPCO facts and figures: Hospice care in America.* Washington, DC: Author.

National Institute for Drug Abuse. (2004). Monitoring the future. *National Institute for Drug Abuse Newsletter.* Washington, DC: Author.

Richmond, M. (1917). *Social diagnosis.* New York: Sage Foundation.

SBIRT. (2007). *Screening, brief intervention, referral and treatment.* U.S. Department of Health and Human Services Substance Abuse and Mental Health Services Administration. Retrieved June 3, 2008, from http://sbirt.samhsa.gov/core_comp/index.htm

Sloan, P., Vanderveer, B., Snapp, J., Johnson, M., & Sloan, D. (1999). Cancer pain assessment and management recommendations by hospice nurses. *Journal of Pain and Symptom Management, 18*(2), 103–110.

Sorocco, K. H., & Ferrell, S. W. (1996). Alcohol use among older adults. *Journal of General Psychology, 133*(4), 453–467.

Substance Abuse and Mental Health Services Administration. (2007). *Tip 26: Substance abuse among older adults* (p. 454). Rockville, MD: Author.

Sue, D., & Sue, D. (2008). *Counseling for cultural diversity* (5th ed.). Hoboken, NJ: Wiley.

Sullivan, P. F., & Myers, J. M. (2005). Alcohol dependence: A validation of diagnosis by interview. *Alcoholism and Experimental Research, 29*(3), 417–432.

Tarzian, A. J., & Hoffman, D. E. (2005). Barriers to managing pain in the nursing home: Findings from a statewide survey. *Journal of the American Medical Directors Association, 6*(3), S:13–S:19.

U.S. Food and Drug Administration. (2001). *2001 Safety alerts for human medical products.* Retrieved June 3, 2008, from www.fda.gov/Safety/MedWatch

Valliant, P., & Pottier, D. (2003). Personality and executive functioning as risk factors in recidivists. *Psychological Reports, 92*(1), 299.

vonGunten, C. F. (2005). Interventions to manage symptoms at the end of life. *Journal of Palliative Medicine, 8*(Suppl.), 1, S88–S94.

Waldorf, D., Reinarman, C., & Murphy, S. (1991). *Cocaine changes: The experience of using and quitting.* Philadelphia, PA: Temple University Press.

Whitbourne, S. (2002). *The aging individual.* New York: Springer Publishing Company.

3

The Physiological, Psychological, and Spiritual Effects of Addiction

Amy was agitated after she learned that her father was starting with hospice. She knew what this meant: As his only daughter, she would be expected to help with his care. That would mean spending more time with him.

All of her life, Amy had done her best to distance herself from her parents. To avoid seeing them drink themselves into a stupor every night, she would come by to visit during the day, but only when she had to. Now there would be no more avoiding. Amy knew that it was her duty to help her mother care for her dying father. And she would do what she could, as willingly as she could. But she saw it as a trial and a test. She didn't have to like it.

Addiction is often described as a *family* disease. There are principally three reasons why this is the case. First, the presence of chemical dependency in one member of the family often has consequences for other members of that family. Among the impacts of addiction are family conflict, depression, anxiety, financial difficulties, legal problems, school or work issues, and various physical problems (Smyth, 1995). Clearly, many families are affected by the psychosocial consequences of addiction.

Second, addiction has physical costs as well. Just as other chronic diseases, such as diabetes and heart disease, have physical consequences on the body, so does addiction. We will discuss these physical effects, and also how the biological markers of addiction can be genetically passed from generation to generation.

Third, addiction is a family disease insofar as it has identifiable *spiritual* effects on family members who are addicts as well as on the persons who would care for or love them. We will define what we mean by spiritual, and describe these effects.

All of these aspects have a combined impact upon the provision of end-of-life care. Each aspect presents its own challenges to hospice teams. Considered together, all three aspects mandate adjustments in how holistic end-of-life care is delivered. To that end, the biological, psychological, sociocultural, and spiritual dimensions of addiction need to be addressed—both for the patient and for the family.

In each of these aspects of addiction, there is a constant tension between the individual and the family or social system. Later (in chapter 4), we will discuss this tension differently, in the context of family systems theory. For now it is sufficient to say that when it comes to addiction, one cannot speak only of the individual or of the family. Instead, in every aspect, *both* the individual and the family need to be taken into account.

PHYSIOLOGICAL ASPECTS OF ADDICTION

The medical model of addiction emphasizes that the addict has no "choice." This lack of choice is the key element in many definitions of addiction. According to Brenda Schaeffer, "for our purposes, we will define addiction as a habit that has gone unconscious; a compulsive ritual that is no longer a choice; a psychological or physical attachment to an object, often characterized by withdrawal, or intensity of symptoms, when the object is removed" (Schaeffer, 1997, p. 7). (The concept of "object attachment" will be discussed further in chapter 5.)

Both of the alternative models discussed in chapter 2—the moral model and the behavioral model—posit that the addict makes choices, and thus is responsible for his or her behavior. According to those models, addictive behavior could be corrected by either reward or punishment, or by sheer acts of will. These models posit that an addict has the ability to stop—if he or she wants to stop.

However, following the disease model, we can understand why neither incentives nor punishments fully work as correctives to the addict's behavior. Substance use, misuse, and abuse, combined with a genetic predisposition to becoming addicted, effectively rob the addict of free will—or at least impair the addict to the degree that the addict is unable to stop. In this way, the addict cannot be completely responsible for his or her behavior.

> Since the 1960s, we have seen the development of an awareness of addiction as a chronic relapsing and potentially fatal disease with the target organ being the brain. The disease of addiction is an interplay of genetic and environmental factors, in which the compulsive addiction to psychoactive drugs has a neurological basis. From the medical point of view, addiction can be viewed as a chronic disease similar to diabetes.... Unfortunately for many, the societal view of addiction has focused on behavior of the addict rather than a dysfunction of the brain. (Smith & Heilig, 2004, p. 13)

An emphasis on the lack of choice can be seen in definitions of the term: "Addiction is an unconscious, bio-chemical process" (Haroutunian, 2008). It is "not only a brain disease, but also a biological, psychological, social and spiritual disease ... an incurable, chronic and progressive disease prone to relapse" (Davis, 2008).

The paradox of the disease is that continued substance use is self-destructive. Far from promoting survival, addiction undermines health. Yet the mechanisms in the brain that stimulate drug craving can remain active even after the addict has been in recovery. The medical view of addiction is "a chronic relapsing and potentially fatal disease with the target organ being the brain" (Smith & Heilig, 2004, p. 13), which suggests that when choices are to be made, they are limited to the disease itself.

Once it is understood that addiction is chronic and potentially fatal, we can see addiction as being analogous to other chronic diseases, such as diabetes and heart disease. All have certain biological bases and genetic predispositions. For all, the treatment goal is not so much to cure the disease; rather, the goal is to *manage* the disease so that it is no longer life-threatening. When treatment is pursued in this way, it is possible for addicts to regain control of their lives. And for hospice professionals, it may be easier to understand addiction as a challenge to pain and symptom management.

There is an added challenge to addiction at the end of life. Hospice professionals can help patients and families understand the terminal trajectories of different diseases. However, functional decline varies considerably at the end of life, making preparation for the dying process difficult (Chen, Chan, Kiely, Morris, & Mitchell, 2007). Because of the complications that addiction imposes on physiological functioning, the normal disease trajectories that are familiar to end-of-life care professionals may be even less clear.

Comorbidities and Metabolic Changes

Once diagnostic determination of addiction is made, it is useful to look at the other biological impacts of addiction. There is a preponderance of research studies on the impact of alcohol addiction. Alcohol is known to have direct toxic, systemic, and biochemical/nutritional effects, and it contributes to various cancers (Krawiec, Cylwik, Chrostek, Supronowicz, & Szmitkowski, 2008). Colorectal cancer, for example, is associated with high alcohol consumption (Toriola, Kurl, Laukanen, Mazengo, & Kauhanen, 2008). Addiction to both nicotine and alcohol is common, and the combined use contributes significantly to head and neck cancers (Miller & Gold, 1998). Tobacco and alcohol are principal risk factors for cancers of the mouth, pharynx, and larynx (Righini, Karkas, Morei, Soriano, & Reyt, 2008).

Alcohol abuse also causes changes in blood concentrations of lipids, believed to increase the risk of cardiovascular disease (Krawiec, Cylwik, Chrostek, Supronowicz, & Szmitkowski, 2008). Alcohol is toxic to the development of red blood cells; heavy users may exhibit high blood pressure, irregular heart rhythms, enlarged liver or spleen, and neuropathy (DiMartini, 2004). Malnourishment is often present in those who have chronic alcohol abuse, as a result of reduced nutritional intake or because of alcohol's direct effect on absorption (Cortes, 2008). Alcohol dependence is also associated with more severe neurocognitive changes noted with increased age (Durazzo, Rothlind, Gazdzinski, & Meyerhoff, 2008). Widespread cerebral atrophy is found in patients addicted to alcohol (Mechtachcheriakov et al., 2007). Women's health is disproportionately compromised by excess alcohol consumption, as women are more vulnerable to the effects of alcohol than men, and more likely to suffer poor nutrition and anemia (Jordan & Franklin, 2003).

Addiction to other drugs is associated with many chronic and debilitating conditions (Liberto & Oslin, 1997). For example, addiction is frequently a co-occurring disorder with cardiovascular disease, stroke, cancer, HIV/AIDS, liver diseases (including Hepatitis B and C), lung disease, obesity, and mental disorders. Other drugs can also be toxic to the heart, brain, and digestive organs. Hypertension, hepatitis C, and psychiatric disorders are frequent comorbidities with all forms of addiction (Durazzo, Rothlind, Gazdzinski, & Meyerhoff, 2008).

Finally, substance use and abuse can contribute to many mental health and behavioral disorders. Alcohol and drug addiction are leading risk factors in suicide and suicidal behavior (Miller, Giannini, & Gold, 1992). Addiction alters mental status and can exacerbate pre-existing mental illnesses (Miller, 1989; Terenius, 1996; Zakrzewski & Hector, 2004). Substance abuse also increases the risk of family violence (Murphy & O'Farrell, 1997), and marital problems (Wakefield, Williams, Yost, & Patterson, 1996).

As discussed in chapter 2, many older adults with one or more of the common co-morbidities are never assessed for alcohol and/or drug abuse; thus the underlying addiction may never be identified. Perhaps for hospice and end-of-life professionals, addiction is best understood by looking backwards; that is, assessing past substance use or abuse, as well as current consequences which may derive from that behavior. Only in this way can lifelong patterns of addiction be separated from other aspects of health throughout the life course.

Seldom is an addict alone in suffering the negative health effects of addiction. Those who care for addicted persons are also challenged in many ways. Such stressors can themselves be detrimental to health (Zarit, Stephens, Townsend, & Greene, 1997).

Pain and Symptom Management

The detrimental biological effects of addiction and other diseases that often accompany it lead to a constellation of challenges for those who provide end-of-life care for addicts and their families.

First, in most cases the body's metabolism has been altered by addiction, and not merely in ways that are manifested in the disease whose diagnosis has brought the person to end-of-life care. The physical alterations of addiction, especially the impact on the liver as well as an increased tolerance of drugs, lead to complications in the relief of physical pain. *Clearance* (the rate at which toxic substances are eliminated by the kidneys and liver) is likely to be slowed due to the damage caused by addiction. Because of slower metabolic and clearance mechanisms, addicts and former addicts who have become terminal patients are more likely to experience adverse drug and alcohol interactions.

This creates certain specific issues related to end-of-life care, where careful administration of pain medication, in particular, must be adjusted to maintain a constant level of pain control. For the addict, the ability to expel toxic substances may take longer. Thus, typically prescribed dosages may not be sufficient to manage pain, yet may have more toxic effects.

Second, since chemical dependency is a brain disease, and since alterations in brain functioning bring about an addict's craving, the *desire* for medications is manifested differently in the addict than in the nonaddict. Addicts not in recovery may exhibit a craving for more medications. There is also the question of how accurately they will report pain; addicted patients may seek more medication by misreporting the amount of pain they feel. Hospice teams rely on patients to report their pain accurately; thus the traditional practice in end-of-life care is to believe the patient, and scale pain as he or she does. However, when it comes to treating an addict, the question arises: Can the addict be believed? Pain management practices often promote *self*-administration of medications, whenever possible. This usually empowering practice takes on a different meaning when an addict is the patient. Families and professionals therefore often struggle with how (or whether) to allow the addict to self-administer pain medication.

Addicts in recovery, on the other hand, may be reluctant to take medications from which they might otherwise find relief—for fear of jeopardizing their recovery. They may fear self-administration of pain medication as making it too easy to relapse. Since this is a self-image issue as well as a medical one, this ambivalence is no small matter for end-of-life care professionals. However, it may be helpful for such patients to know that it is well established that use of pain-relieving drugs does not cause addiction in patients who are dying and being treated for pain (NHPCO, 2007).

The request (or refusal) of pain medication may also reactivate certain family dynamics. The addict may want more medication than is typically prescribed; or the family may want to keep the addict from receiving any medications at all.

Third, persons and families with histories of addiction have differing relationships to pain and the medications used to relieve it. Addiction often brings about a familiarity with controlled substances the average nonaddict does not have. For an addict, the euphoria that ensues from an abused substance becomes its own trigger for continued use and abuse. In addition, the families themselves will have already adapted to the presence of pain and suffering—and to the substances used to relieve them. Often they frame this adaptation in pseudomedical terms; they might say, for example, that the addict is "self-medicating." In other words, the family and the addict will have already organized themselves around pain (Bushfield, 2006), in recognizable ways. By the time the addict comes to end-of-life care, pain may have already become a predominating presence within the family.

A fourth aspect is that there may be more than one addict in the family (either in the patient's home, or in the extended family). Since most hospice care is provided at home (National Hospice and Palliative Care Organization, 2007), with a family member serving as primary caregiver, there is a question of whether caregivers or others in the family can be trusted with controlled substances. Considering that approximately 6.2 million Americans abuse prescription drugs (often opioids and painkillers) (Smith & Heilig, 2004, p.15), we can see that the use of controlled substances in the home could present temptations to addicted family members. For this reason, assessing for addiction among family caregivers would be best end-of-life care practice, and hospice physicians should be cautious when prescribing adequate medications.

In many families with histories of addiction, there can be active addicts and addicts in varying states of recovery. The *temptation* of having controlled substances available is an aspect of end-of-life care that professionals should address.

Basic principles and guidelines have been developed for prescribing controlled substances to terminally ill patients with addiction (Kirsh & Passik, 2006). These guidelines are supported by many of our premises regarding end-of-life care for those with histories of addiction. Most hospice professionals would likely be familiar with one aspect of these guidelines, with respect to prescribing. Kirsh and Passik suggest that close monitoring and more frequent visits may be required, and that

Exhibit 3.1

Basic Principles for Prescribing Controlled Substances to Patients With Advanced Illness and Issues of Addiction

Choose an opioid based on around-the-clock dosing.

Choose long-acting agents when possible.

As much as possible, limit or eliminate the use of short-acting or "break-through" doses.

Use nonopioid adjuvants when possible and monitor for compliance with those medications.

Use nondrug adjuvants whenever possible (i.e., relaxation techniques, distraction, biofeedback, TNS, communication about thoughts and feelings of pain).

If necessary, limit the amount of medication given at any one time (i.e., write prescriptions for a few days' worth or a weeks' worth of medication at a time).

Utilize pill counts and urine toxicology screens as necessary.

If compliance is suspect or poor, refer to an addictions specialist.

Source: Kirsh, K., & Passik, S. (2006). Palliative care of the terminally ill drug addict. *Cancer Investigations, 24*, 427.

small quantities of drugs be prescribed, with no renewals given if appointments are missed or if home supplies are not accounted for. Any changes to dosages must be carefully reviewed and approved (Kirsh & Passik, p. 429). Exhibit 3.1 summarizes some of these guidelines.

Perhaps less familiar to all hospice professionals are the authors' additional recommendations for: (a) the use of a multidisciplinary approach, (b) thorough assessment of substance-abuse history, (c) the need to recognize specific drug-abuse behaviors, and (d) the essential use of family sessions and meetings (Kirsh & Passik, 2006).

PSYCHOSOCIAL ASPECTS OF ADDICTION

We will now examine some essential elements of the *psychosocial* aspects of addiction: family roles, rules, and relationships. These concepts have become part of the psychology of the addict and the addict's family.

Some of these concepts can be descriptive of life in a family where one or more persons are chemically dependent. Thus, these concepts also describe the social environment within which the addict lives. Because these concepts are experienced both internally in the addict's psyche *and* externally in the social environment, we discuss them together as psychosocial aspects of addiction.

Issues related to addiction influence all behavior within families (Lederer, 1991). The psychosocial aspects of addiction tend to persist throughout the life of the addict and the family. Often at the end of the life of one of the family members, these psychosocial aspects are amplified, even as the impending death of a family member threatens to change the ways that the family members interact. Addressing family relationships without acknowledging the impact of addiction only serves to foster continuing patterns, which likely will not be useful to family functioning (Treadway, 1989), especially at the end of life.

We believe it is useful to examine the three key areas—family roles, rules, and relationships—endemic to family functioning because all family systems are governed by roles and rules that have typically been developed and modified within the family relationships over time (Andreae, 1996). In the following sections, we will explore the impact that both terminal illness and addiction might have on each of these key areas.

Family Roles

Much of the literature on families and addiction focuses on the roles that other family members play in maintaining addiction. These roles are patterns of interaction, and are influenced by both the expectations family members have of each other, and by whether or not family members meet those expectations (Andreae, 1996). For example, if an addict exhibits extreme behavior, such as passing out each night after drinking, there is likely another member of the family who develops another extreme behavior (such as secrecy, or covering up the addict's behavior). Both behaviors are reciprocal: one serves to maintain the other, and this is common in families with addiction (Treadway, 1989). Within families, each member develops his or her role based, in part, on what others expect of them; whether or not they feel competent to fulfill the expectation; and whether or not the expectations are ambiguous (Andreae, 1996). In this context, conflicts may develop as, on occasion, what is expected of someone in one role conflicts with what is expected of the family member in another role. Thus, families are continually changing and adapting. However, many families struggle with restructuring and coping, and in families with addiction, these struggles are likely to result in more rigid roles and rules (Minuchin & Fishman, 1981).

This interpretation suggests that there are certain predictable roles that are re-enacted in families experiencing addiction, and we present a sampling of them here, but with the following word of caution: These roles, and the names used to describe them, represent certain *functions* in the family. They are not to be confused with the *identity* of the person taking on that particular function.

One constellation of roles in the chemically dependent family might be (Betty Ford Center, 2008, p. 27):

- **The (Identified) Addict or Addicted Person:** creates the chaos to which everyone else reacts; represents the family "problem"; is inconsistent in responsibility; is self-centered.
- **The Chief Enabler:** as the Rescuer or Martyr, can suffer from physical illness (somatic stress); represents control; is super-responsible but overbearing and out of touch with self.
- **The Family Hero:** does what's right and achieves visible success; is the one of whom the family is proud; but is judgmental of other members.
- **The Scapegoat/Rebel:** the individual's anger-driven defiance takes the focus off the chemically dependent family member—and draws negative attention (in contrast to the family's hero).
- **The Lost Child:** is the withdrawn loner of the family who provides *relief* in that s/he appears to be the one no one else has to worry about; tends to be quiet, with few friends (not a large social network).
- **The Mascot/Clown:** provides fun and humor for the family, but is emotionally fragile and immature; tends to be hyperactive.

We can perhaps better understand George and Wilma's family if we see them as filling these roles:

- **George:** the "identified addict."

■ **Wilma (wife):** the "chief enabler."
■ **John (the son, with his own history of substance abuse):** the "mascot/clown," because of how he made his parents laugh and the "scapegoat," because of how he disappointed his parents with his own substance abuse—in spite of now being in recovery.
■ **Amy (the daughter):** the "lost child" because of how she withdrew from the family's interactions; and the "hero," for remaining sober, for having a stable marriage, and for her judgments about how the rest of the family behaves.

Roles can change as families evolve and people age. After John grew into adulthood for example, and his parents began to acknowledge his drinking problem—their roles may have changed, which is something that they never acknowledged to themselves. Here is how they each may have become identified after George entered hospice:

■ **John:** the "identified addict";
■ **George:** the "scapegoat," knowing how his children (and his wife, tacitly) blamed him for the state of things in the family;
■ **Wilma:** still the "chief enabler";
■ **Amy:** the hero, but she might also be less aware in her adulthood how her childhood as the "lost child" still influenced her behaviors and her feelings about herself and the other members of her family.

Rules

Every family structures and governs itself by rules, many of which are unstated (Andreae, 1996). Rules usually serve to help family members determine what is permitted and what is forbidden, and they develop in connection with the roles and behaviors others in the family display (Andreae, 1996). We believe that families with histories of addiction can be characterized by their tendency to be more rule-based because of their more rigid adherence to the roles mentioned earlier. These rules are not likely expressed aloud; rather, they tend to be tacitly lived out. And in families with addiction, these rules are developed within a context of reciprocal extremes of behavior (according to polarized roles, above) and an absence of a model of normalcy (Fossum & Mason, 1986).

The reason why families with histories of addiction tend to be more rule-based than families without such a history has to do with the role that *power* plays in such families. Control over others substitutes for self-control, and power substitutes for love. (See the section on spirituality later in this chapter.) From a nonfamily systems perspective, control issues arise because of the unconscious and suppressed fears in families with histories of addiction (Schaeffer, 1997, p. 77f), but we may also see how, within the drive for stability, that power and control (overfunctioning) may exist in concert with another's underfunctioning. The power imbalances created in these families is often highly reactive (Lederer, 1991).

Three common rules in families with histories of addiction are: Don't Talk, Don't Feel, and Don't Trust.

■ **Don't Talk:** In this rule is the origin of the family's secret keeping—toward those outside the family, as well as for those inside the family. Family members are discouraged (and even ordered) not to talk about specific behaviors that they observe in one another.

The rule of "don't talk" will likely limit the information that end-of-life professionals might gain from a family, about themselves or each other. Hospice professionals, many of whom are quite sensitive to those in their care, may sense a family's reticence and simply continue to avoid topics which, when broached, receive a cool reception. Thus, hospice professionals unwittingly become part of the conspiracy of silence.

■ **Don't Feel:** In fact, this rule is more about what to feel and what not to feel. That is, family members are supposed to feel proud of the family and happy to be a part of it. At the same time, family members should not cry, feel sad, or be angry. Thus some feelings are ruled in—and others are ruled out.

The rule of "don't feel" may particularly confuse family members as one of them dies, a time which is usually fraught with feeling. Children who grow up in such families often have significant confusion about what they do feel; it becomes difficult to recognize an authentic emotion after many years of substituting approved and acceptable emotions for that which was actually felt.

■ **Don't Trust:** This rule is as much about the atmosphere within the family as about not trusting any specific person outside of it. One aspect of the lack of trust in families with histories of addiction has to do with how they come to regard each other. This is related to the relative lack of safety or security felt within the family (see the section on "boundaries" below). But it also has to do with how one is taught to regard people *outside* the family. If one *is not* allowed to talk or feel, then one *does* become distrustful—both of others and of one's self. What if someone were to speak out about the addiction or to express his or her true feelings? The potential that the truth about the family's life might be exposed creates its own distrust.

Distrust in families with histories of addiction is a prudent caution. One cannot trust authority figures. One cannot trust that someone who is helpful or caring has no other motive than the one that is professed. We can see how this attitude may present problems to end-of-life professionals, who seek to be trusted by a family—and yet may be persistently regarded with suspicion.

This atmosphere of mistrust and suspicion has other emotional effects upon the people living in it, especially upon the children growing up in it. Family members learn about shame and blame—who is to be ashamed and why, and who is or is not to blame. For example, from their parents, the children might learn: "If I teach you not to trust, and I let you down, don't blame me!" Or, if children expected to get something from their parents—and didn't—it was said to be the *children's* fault. "Fault finding" is a well-honed skill in families with histories of addiction.

Our point is that each of these areas of family life—roles, rules, and relationships—overlap and influence each other. Because we learn our first lessons about how to relate to others and how to conduct ourselves in relationships from our families, we can readily understand how those lessons may be quite different in families with histories of addiction.

Relationships

There are three aspects of relationships among members of families with histories of addiction that we will highlight because of their saliency in end-of-life care: denial, boundaries, and losses (Anderson, 1989; Carter & McGoldrick, 1988; Franklin, 2003; Goldstein, 1981; Jordan & Munson, 2000; Rosen, 1990; Yesavage et al., 1983).

Denial

Denial is the capacity to frame one's perspective and interpret one's circumstances in such a way that significant aspects of reality are omitted or minimized. Denial is most often used as a psychological defense, against feeling overwhelmed or against experiencing anxiety, for example. But it can also become a habit, a point of view of omission instead of inclusion. In denial, even though we perceive or recognize something, we may not accept it (Goldstein, 1996).

Families with histories of addiction can be characterized by the pervasiveness of denial among their members. What began perhaps as a way of *coping* with a problem or stress has become characteristic of their perspectives, and thus an explanation of their behaviors. Minimization and/or wishful thinking function as aspects of denial. Thus members of these families tend to be reactive—often reacting more slowly to the challenges of end-of-life care. For instance, they may wait longer than other families to initiate hospice care; they may balk at instituting changes in their way of life or adapting to new necessities; and they may resist suggestions or even requirements made by the hospice team. Often the family members' resistance, minimization, or denial, simply do not make sense to the hospice team. Their behavior may seem irrational or nonsensical to the hospice team—but will seem perfectly reasonable to the family members themselves.

For example, denial may arise in issues involving the administration of pain medications—families may advocate either overmedicating or (more commonly) undermedicating, with the result that the person dying is in more pain than seems reasonable to the hospice team. Yet, when challenged to administer more, the family member may deny the pain of the dying person, often by saying that they do not wish to make them an addict or reactivate their addiction.

Boundaries

Boundaries have to do with the invisible but important borders around us that help us define who we are and what we have. Our personal boundaries vary with each of us, and fluctuate, depending on our vulnerability, experiences, ability to be intimate, and our consistency of self. But others' respect for our boundaries is necessary to our self-respect. Boundaries permit integrity and dignity.

The lack of healthy separations among family members and the chronic and persistent disrespect of each other's space characterize families with histories of addiction and make it difficult for family members to have separate identities. Boundary violations not only lead to higher instances of abusive behavior and violence, but they also lead to overidentification with others—a sense that "you cut yourself and I bleed."

Lack of boundaries may become especially problematic in the provision of end-of-life care, particularly because home hospice itself often challenges boundaries, even when they are healthfully established. For example, children may be called upon to care for parents, even those of the opposite gender. These circumstances are challenging enough in the best of relational circumstances. But when there has been a history of permeable or nonexistent boundaries, then it can become all the more difficult to establish appropriate boundaries during end-of-life care. Histories of fears and resentments can arise—and may, but more likely may *not*, be voiced (following the "Don't Speak" rule).

Hospice professionals should realize that an addict will likely *not* respect boundaries in order to obtain his/her drug of choice. Addicts behave in the ways that they do simply because they are trying to survive—irrespective of and without regard for another's boundaries or feelings.

Losses

In families with histories of addiction, losses are a matter of course. As an Al-Anon Family Group book states, "Living with alcoholism can feel like we're in a constant state of mourning" (Al-Anon, 2007, p. 23).

Families with histories of addiction are likely to experience a multiplicity of losses, because addiction co-exists with social indicators such as loss of jobs, marital dysfunction, and divorce (Miller, Gold, & Klahr, 1990). The families are not likely to have mourned these losses well, due in part to the "don't talk" and "don't feel" rules mentioned earlier. In fact, individual family members may have adjusted themselves to be emotionally or even geographically far from the family cluster simply in order (consciously or unconsciously) to handle the losses suffered by the family. Thus, when a family member is dying—representing yet another loss—it may not be easy for family members to respond. We will address this topic more thoroughly in chapter 7. For the moment, we acknowledge that losses and grieving those losses—or not—permeates relationships among families with histories of addiction to a degree not experienced by families without such histories.

These three rules can have an impact on how family members are esteemed by end-of-life professionals. Hospice team members may have certain judgments about family members who make themselves available to participate in end-of-life care—and those who do not. In a family with a history of addiction, proximity of family members is not in itself a measure of health. And failure to rise to the occasion of providing help in home hospice care is not in itself an indication of emotional detachment or not caring.

SPIRITUAL ASPECTS OF ADDICTION

Often, the most surprising aspect of recovery for many addicts is its essentially *spiritual* nature. Even addicts who may not have previously considered themselves to be religious, or those who have had negative or even abusive experiences of religion, may come to a spiritual understanding of themselves, and indeed of life, through the recovery process.

First, we should distinguish between "being religious" and "being spiritual." By one definition, spirituality "has to do with our ability to make contact with what matters most to us: relationships, emotions, values, and aspirations. Organized religion is most helpful when it contributes to a person's experience of these deep-seated aspects of one's self" (Betty Ford Center, 2008, p. 21). 12-Step programs, for example, define themselves as "spiritual," not "religious," in nature, following the perspective of Alcoholics Anonymous' advocacy of recovery as "spiritual growth that comes about through spiritual principles" (Alcoholics Anonymous, 2001, p. 47). When we speak about spirituality here, we mean: *the practiced appreciation of that which makes life meaningful.*

Addicts in recovery learn how to lead more meaningful lives simply by learning what makes life meaningful; this is what makes recovery a "spiritual practice." It is precisely this loss of the sense of what is meaningful—or rather, its misplacement into the object of one's addiction—that is at the spiritual core of the addict's experience in addiction.

We mentioned earlier that addiction is essentially a biological and behavioral paradox: that which the addict craves and pursues out of a drive to survive is precisely that which can bring about the addict's demise. Thus all of the spiritual aspects of addiction have to do with this drive to damage oneself in essential ways. Addiction brings about loss in three of life's key dimensions: personhood, community, and capacity to love. In each dimension, addiction is spiritually diminishing and existentially damaging.

The affirmation that spiritual care is a significant component of hospice care comes from the Medicare Hospice Benefit itself, which recognizes spiritual caregiving as one of the four core disciplines. Moreover, the hospice movement has at its origins the recognition of how important spiritual matters become to those who are coming to the end of their lives. There is an abiding sense in hospice that hospice care *is* spiritual care.

In the practice of spiritual care in hospice, however, there is this inherent tension: On the one hand, the affirmation is made that, in some ways, every hospice professional is a spiritual caregiver. Everyone who brings hospice care to the patient and family—whether nurse or physician, social worker or certified nursing assistant—is supposed to bring an awareness of the spiritual life. Moreover, the persons being served by hospice, be they the patient or a family member could, at any time, with any hospice professional, raise a spiritual concern—one that would need to be addressed in some fashion in the moment. For this reason, it is important for every member of the hospice team to be spiritually astute in her/his care.

On the other hand, the standard hospice team typically includes a spiritual care professional, such as a chaplain. These professionals should be equipped to recognize and address the spiritual issues that arise among families receiving hospice care. When spiritual issues arise with other team members, they are best reported to that professional for further address.

Spiritual issues are universal; concerns such as loss of personhood, community, and capacity to love may arise with anyone, addicts and nonaddicts alike. Although they have special relevance for addicted persons and their families, we believe that learning to address these issues would enhance the spiritual caregiving for patients and families for all hospice professionals.

Loss of Personhood: Damage to Self

George and Wilma's son, John, saw himself as having two lives: One life, when he drank; the other life, since he'd been sober. After 2 years of sobriety, he sometimes wondered who that "other guy" was—the person he became when he was drinking and using. He knew he was the same person; he feared that he was the same person. He took comfort from believing he was different now, somehow.

In addiction, one displaces everything that matters most to oneself with only one thing: The drug of choice. This results in a loss of personhood, both in a figurative and in a literal sense. In spiritual terms, the addict is experiencing the consequences of *idolatry*—a relationship with an object that becomes the most significant relationship in a person's life. To recover a sense of what is spiritually appropriate is to recover one's own humanity, beyond the compulsions of the disease. Moreover, it is to experience in oneself a drive for what is life-giving and not life-taking.

The establishment of any idolatrous relationship brings with it feelings of shame. (We will increasingly address the significance of shame throughout this book, culminating in chapter 10.) For the hospice professional, the shame of idolatry can be addressed with understanding and acceptance, with nonjudgment, and without surprise or otherwise trying to "correct" the attachment. It is the idolatry of addiction that demands the most compassion in spiritual care.

As with every issue of spiritual care, the idolatry of the addict raises idolatrous issues or tendencies in the one who provides spiritual care. Thus, addressing idolatry in the addict means becoming aware of idolatry in oneself—and treating both self and other with compassion for it.

Loss of Community: Damage to One's Connections With Others

Amy was trying to be positive about the Heart of Gold Hospice Team. She would come to her parents' house to meet them; she would be polite and answer their questions. But when Bill, the social worker, asked if she wanted the chaplain to call her, she declined. He tried to explain that the hospice team's chaplain might help her discuss issues of dying and grief, but she found him pushy and declined his offer more firmly. She did not want to discuss her feelings with anyone.

The experience of addiction inevitably leads *away* from "belonging" in a healthy way to family and friends. The idolatry of the addict means that the addict has prioritized the relationship to the drug of choice over relationships with other people. This results in a loss of a sense of community. In spiritual terms, the damage that an addict does to relationships with others leads to an experience of *isolation*.

> Isolation is the legacy of addiction in families. Addicts become walled up with their drug(s) of choice and isolate themselves from intimacy with family. Family members become so habituated to this "business as usual," adaptating to addiction that they become cut off from any meaningful connection with the addict or with each other. (Betty Ford Center, 2008, p. 21)

The isolation of the addict may not seem readily apparent; in fact, many addicts may be surrounded by other addicts. Yet in the course of their addiction, addicts become isolated from others with whom they might have healthy relationships. The experience of being high is one that separates and isolates the addict.

Isolation is why social re-networking and social support are as important as they are to the process of recovery. Most, if not all, rehabilitation programs strongly advise the recovering addict—and family members—to begin a program of participation in a 12-Step group. Very often the addict's recovery depends on this re-establishment of "community," of reliable and caring networks of social support.

The successes of social support groups are attributed to "their understanding of others' experiences [as] part of the human condition" (Griefzu, 1996; Muller & Thompson, 2003). A strong sense of social support and coherence helps mitigate feelings of disenfranchisement and separateness, and helps increase individual perceptions of long-term happiness and hope (Anke & Fugle-Meyer, 2003). Social support networks, which have been identified as promoting health benefits, also cushion the effects of stress, reduce mortality rates, increase the likelihood that the individual will seek help, and assist in developing personal coping abilities (Hurdle, 2001). It has been shown that support networks are particularly important to women (DeFrain, 1986; Hurdle, 2001).

By the time hospice services have come to families with a history of addiction, there has likely been an erosion of a sense of belonging to a greater community among the family members. For many with such histories, their relationships with the community outside their family became strained during periods of addiction. Moreover, they are likely to be ambivalent at best about any feelings of belonging they have toward each other.

The degree of isolation in any family with a history of addiction can be assessed according to the nature of their belonging, both to each other, and to organizations beyond the family. Hospice professionals might think in terms of a continuum of communities. For example, the active addict finds "community" within the network of relationships needed to support his or her substance abuse. By contrast, persons in recovery will have developed a variety of networks of support in the community that are supportive and healing.

Hospice professionals should understand that, in spiritual terms, family members' regard of hospice as either threatening or welcoming turns on levels of isolation in and among the family. Of course, hospice intends to be a support network toward healing. This may or may not be regarded by family members as a good thing.

Loss of Love: Damage to One's Significant Relationships

After George came onto hospice service, Wilma began having thoughts and feelings she never had before. One night, as she lay awake, she found herself wondering: Did George really love her? She couldn't remember the last time he'd said it—or the last time she felt it.

She woke George. While he was still groggy, Wilma said to him, "George, do you love me?" George shook his head in annoyance and disbelief. "Of course I love you!" he said, and rolled over with his back to her. At that moment, Wilma did not feel loved at all.

Another spiritual consequence of an addict's idolatry is the damage it does to one's ability to be close in significant relationships. Not only is there a generalized experience of isolation, but there is also a specific impairment of one-on-one relationships. Since the primary relationship is with one's drug of choice, every other relationship has a lower priority. The result is a loss of an ability to love; other values, such as power and control, are embraced.

In other words, addiction impairs one's capacity for *intimacy*. Indeed, one could say that intimacy is a co-casualty of addiction—or even the other way around. For, more often than not, it is not that the capacity for intimacy is lost *after* one becomes an addict. Instead, more than likely, the loss of the capacity for intimacy occurred long before one actually became an addict. For instance, many addicts have histories that include experiences of boundary violations such as abuse or incest (Barrett, 1986; Covington, 1982; McGoldrick, Anderson, & Walsh, 1989; Wilsnack & Beckman, 1984). Such experiences could easily damage many addicts' capacity for intimacy, and foster a need for control. Feeling the chaos in which their lives are immersed, they often use substances out of desire to have some control over something—and thus to seek control over others, even as they fear others' control over them. One definition of an addict could simply be someone who is "intimacy impaired." (See Schaeffer [1997] for an excellent study on intimacy, addiction, and the difference between relationships based on power and control and those based in love.)

Recovery is spiritual in that it restores to the individual the possibility of genuine relationships with others, both in terms of experiences of community, and in terms of authentic intimacy (Schaeffer, 2007). Recovery is, as much as anything, the recovery of the capacity to love.

What this means to the hospice professional providing care to a family with a history of addiction is that they are more likely to observe relationships based on power than love in such families. Hospice professionals may unwittingly find themselves in power struggles with family caregivers over how much medication to give, for instance, when and how often, or in disagreements about what the caregivers report the patient is experiencing as opposed to what is observed and assessed by the hospice professional.

Hospice professionals can help themselves and the families they are serving by remembering two things. First, that what they are observing has been going on in that family's life since before the hospice team arrived—and is likely to continue in one form or another after the hospice team leaves. Therefore, avoiding power struggles with family members whenever possible would be advisable; yet seeing them for what they are when they do arise is even more valuable. Second, since family members are going to be intimacy-challenged or intimacy-impaired, hospice team members would do well to model among themselves relationships with more appropriate and caring boundaries. This means, among other things, working together to overcome "alliances" that family members are likely to make that "split" team members or pit them against each other.

Above all, end-of-life care professionals do well to remember that the dying of one family member inevitably draws other family members closer together. In families with histories of addiction, this can be a very mixed experience. If the end of life is itself an "intimate" time, then this intimacy is likely to be particularly challenging for members of families with histories of addiction.

SUMMARY: TOWARD UNDERSTANDING THE ADDICT AND FAMILY

One of the things to remember in providing end-of-life care for a family with a history of addiction is that one or more of the addictions may be continuing in the course of hospice care. Family members may continue to drink or use drugs—or, for example, may resume smoking, as George did. End-of-life medications may be stolen and used or sold.

Providing end-of-life care is not in itself a mandate for intervention, and end-of-life care professionals have not been sought out by the family to be their therapists (at least in regard to addiction). Thus the hospice professional can find himself or herself, even in the best of circumstances, in the rather strange position of being able to identify addiction behaviors but being powerless to address them within the framework of end-of-life care.

Still, there are things the end-of-life care professional can do. Coming into such families with a greater awareness of who they are and why they function the way they do may lead to a greater understanding and appreciation of them which they might not otherwise have received. This understanding and acceptance can be, in itself, healing.

By the same token, it is unwise and perhaps unfair for hospice teams to expect these families to adjust to hospice's standard ways of proceeding. It is better that hospice teams adjust their procedures, so as not to tempt or otherwise disrespect the families under their care. For instance, perhaps medications should not be left in the home, but rather brought as scheduled and administered by a nurse or another team member. Also, levels of trustworthiness and appropriate boundary establishment, for example, cannot simply be presumed.

Above all, awareness of addiction, its nature, and its consequences is meant to guide end-of-life care professionals in their provision of care to *all* persons. In their endeavor to preserve dignity at a time in life when dignity is most threatened, end-of-life care professionals may find that it is not only the dignity of the dying that needs their attention, but the dignity of everyone in the family as well.

REFERENCES

Al-Anon Family Groups. (2007). *Opening our hearts, transforming our losses.* Virginia Beach, VA: Author.

Alcoholics Anonymous. (2001). *Alcoholics anonymous* (4th ed.). New York: Alcoholics Anonymous World Services.

Anderson, C. (1989).Women and serious mental disorders. In M. McGoldrick, C. Anderson, & F. Walsh (Eds.), *Women in families* (pp. 381–405). New York: W. W. Norton.

Andreae, D. (1996). Systems theory and social work treatment. In F. J. Turner (Ed.), *Social work treatment* (pp. 601–616). New York: Columbia University Press.

Anke, A., & Fugl-Meyer, A. (2003). Life satisfaction several years after severe multiple trauma: A retrospective investigation. *Clinical Rehabilitation, 17,* 431–442.

Bushfield, S. (2006). Pain and the family. In M. V. Boswell & B. E. Cole (Eds.), *Weiner's pain management: A guide for clinicians* (7th ed., pp. 61–65). Boca Raton, FL: CRC Press.

Betty Ford Center. (2008). *Family programs work book.* Rancho Mirage, CA: Author.

Carter, B., & McGoldrick, M. (1989). *The changing family life cycle: A framework for family therapy.* Boston: Allyn & Bacon.

Chen, J., Chan, D., Kiely, D., Morris, J., & Mitchell, S. (2007). Terminal trajectories of functional decline in the long-term care setting. *Journals of Gerontology,* Series A, 62, 531–536.

Corcoran, M., & Barrett, K. (1991). Environmental influences on behavior of elderly. *Journal of Physical and Occupational Therapy in Geriatrics, 11,* 131–152.

Cortes, M. (2008). Nutrition and chronic alcohol abuse. *Nutricion Hospitaliaria, 23* (2), 3–7.

Covington, S. (1982). *Sexual experience, dysfunction and abuse: A comparative study of alcoholic and non-alcoholic women.* Doctoral dissertation, Union Graduate School, Cincinnati, OH.

Davis, S. (2008). *The disease of addiction: Definitions of addiction* (DVD #S7277). Rancho Mirage, LA: Betty Ford Center.

DeFrain, J. (1986). *Stillborn: The invisible death*. Lexington, MA: Rowman & Littlefield.

DiMartini, A. (2008). *A clinical guide to assessing alcohol use and problems*. Pittsburgh, PA: Alcohol Medical Scholars Program.

Durazzo, T., Rothlind, J., Gazdzinski, S., & Meyerhoff, D. (2008). The relationship of socio-demographic factors, medical, psychiatric and substance-misuse co-morbidities to neurocognition in short term abstinent alcohol-dependent individuals. *Alcohol, 42*(6), 439–449.

Fossum, M. A., & Mason, M. J. (1986). *Facing shame: Families in recovery*. New York: W. W. Norton.

Goldstein, E. (1981). *Promoting competence in clients: A new/old approach to social work practice*. New York: Free Press.

Goldstein, E. (1996). Ego psychology theory. In F. J. Turner (Ed.), *Social work treatment* (pp. 191–217). New York: Free Press.

Griefzu, S. (1996). Grieving families need your help. *RN, 58*(9), 22.

Haroutunian, H. L. (2008). *The disease of addiction: Disease in balance* (DVD #S7276). Rancho Mirage, CA: Betty Ford Center.

Hurdle, D. (2001). Social support: A critical factor in women's health and health promotion. *Health and Social Work, 26*(2), 72–79.

Jordan, C., & Franklin, C. (2003). *Clinical assessment for social workers*. Chicago: Lyceum Books.

Kirsh, K. L., & Passik, S. D. (2006). Palliative care of the terminally ill drug addict. *Cancer Investigations, 24*, 425–431.

Krawiec, A., Cylwik, B., Chrostek, L., Supronowicz, Z., & Szmitkowski, M. (2008). The effect on chronic alcohol abuse on lipids, lipoproteins, and apolipoproteins concentration. *Polski Merkuriusz Lekarski, 24*(144), 521–525.

Lederer, G. S. (1991). Alcohol in the family system. In F. Herz-Brown (Ed.), *Reweaving the family tapestry* (pp. 219–241). New York: W.W. Norton.

Liberto, J., & Oslin, D. (1995). Older adults misuse of alcohol, medicines, and other drugs. *Research and Practice Issues, 13*, 94–112.

McGoldrick, M., Anderson, C., & Walsh, F. (1989). *Women in families: A framework for family therapy*. New York: W. W. Norton.

Mechtachcheriakov, S., Brenneis, C., Egger, K., Koppelstaetter, F., Schocke, M., & Marksteiner, J. (2007). A widespread pattern of cerebral atrophy in patients with alcohol addiction revealed by voxel-based morphometry. *Journal of Neurology, Neurosurgery & Psychiatry, 78*(6), 610–614.

Miller, N. S. (1989). *Comprehensive handbook of drug and alcohol addiction*. New York: Marcel Dekker.

Miller, N. S., Giannini, A. J., & Gold, M. S. (1992). Suicide risk associated with drug and alcohol addiction. *Cleveland Clinic Journal of Medicine, 59*(5), 535–538.

Miller, N. S., & Gold, M. S. (1998). Co-morbid cigarette and alcohol addiction: Epidemiology and treatment. *Journal of Addictive Diseases, 17*(1), 55–66.

Miller, N. S., Gold, M. S., & Klahr, A. L. (1990). Diagnosis of addiction. *Substance Use and Misuse, 25*(7), 735–744.

Minuchin, S., & Fishman, H. (1981). *Family therapy techniques*. Cambridge, MA: Harvard University Press.

Muller, E. E., & Thompson, C. L. (2003). The experience of grief after bereavement: A phenomenological study. *Journal of Mental Health Counseling, 25*(3), 183–195.

Murphy, C., & O'Farrell, T. J. (1997). Couple communication patterns of maritally aggressive and nonaggressive male alcoholics. *Journal of Studies on Alcohol, 58,* 34–51.

National Hospice and Palliative Care Organization. (2007). *NHPCO facts and figures: Hospice care in America.* Washington, DC: Author.

Righini, C., Karkas, A., Morei, N., Soriano, E., & Reyt, E. (2008). Risk factors for cancer of the oral cavity, pharynx and larynx. *Presse Medicale, 37*(9), 1229–1240.

Rosen, E . J. (1991). Families facing terminal illness. In F. Brown (Ed.), *Reweaving the family tapestry* (pp. 262–285). New York: W.W. Norton.

Schaeffer, B. (1997). *Is it love or is it addiction?* Center City, MN: Hazelden.

Smith, D. & Heilig, S, (2004). Addiction as a brain disease: Methamphetamine as a case study. *San Francisco Medicine, 77*(5), 13–15.

Terenius, L. (1996). Naloxone treatment in depression. *Journal of Orthopsychiatry, 53,* 576–594.

Toriola, A. T., Kurl, S., Laukanen, J., Mazengo, C., & Kauhanen, J. (2008). Alcohol consumption and risk of colorectal cancer. *European Journal of Epidemiology, 23* (6), 395–401.

Treadway, D. (1989). *The healing journey through addiction.* New York: John Wiley.

Wakefield, P. J., Williams, R. E., Yost, E. B., & Patterson, K. M. (1996). *Couple therapy for alcoholism: A cognitive-behavioral treatment manual.* New York: Guilford Press.

Wilsnack, S., & Beckman, L. (1984). *Alcohol problems in women: Antecedents, consequences, and intervention.* New York: Guilford Press.

Yesavage, J., Brink, T., Rose, T., Lum, O., Huang, V., Adey, M., et al. (1983). Development and validation of a geriatric depression screening scale: A preliminary report. *Journal of Psychiatric Research, 17,* 37–49.

Zakrzewski, R. F., & Hector, M. H. (2004). The lived experience of alcohol addiction: Men of AA. *Issues in Mental Health Nursing, 25*(1), 61–77.

Zarit, S., Stephens, M., Townsend, A., & Green, R. (1998). Stress reduction for family caregivers: Effects of adult day care use. *Journals of Gerontology Series B Psychological Sciences and Social Sciences, 53B*(5), S267–277.

4

A Systems Approach to Dying: What Every Hospice Team Needs to Know About Family Systems Theory

George walked slowly out to the backyard through the French doors, and shuffled toward the Adirondack chair with the ashtray on one armrest and the pack of cigarettes on the other. He settled himself and lit up. He closed his eyes, fought the anxiety that came from being short of breath, and told himself that it felt good just to be able to enjoy his cigarettes again.

From inside the house, Wilma and Amy watched him. Amy's face twisted in pique, "How can you stand it, Mother? Watching him kill himself like that?" Wilma shrugged. "He says he enjoys it," she said. "And there's not much else he does." She paused, and added, "Soon he won't even be able to do that...." Her voice trailed off, leading them both to contemplate that coming day in silence.

Families are our primary relationships. What we learn about ourselves and others—how to relate, how to get along, how to be together—always comes first from the families in which we were raised.

Hospice is also about relationships. For hospice professionals to be proficient at what they do, they have to be able to establish strong working relationships with the wide variety of family members whom they meet—and with each other, as members of the hospice team. Being relationally adept is a prerequisite for anyone seeking to become a hospice professional.

This is important because it prioritizes a skill that is often over-looked. Within the medical field, it is often said that "hospice care is comfort care"—in other words, hospice is an extension of the pain-relieving specialty known as palliative care. Certainly, this is one aspect of hospice, and hospice professionals are, generally speaking, quite skilled at palliative care and pain abatement. People who can do this well are valued, of course. But such people may or may not be skilled in *relationships*.

A focus on relationships widens the scope of care in two ways. First, the emphasis shifts from focusing primarily on the individual who is dying to one that includes the family or other participants in the system of care. Without taking into account the *system* in which the dying person is living, and the cooperation and motivations of other persons in that system, palliation is simply less effective than it might otherwise be.

Moreover, a focus that emphasizes relationships will better illumi-nate the relationship that the dying person has with his or her own pain. Sometimes, for example, with all other meaningful measures of being alive having been lost—a dying person will prefer a certain level of pain simply because it reminds him that he is still alive. Feeling pain may be preferred to feeling nothing. Palliative efforts may be frustrated simply because this relationship is underappreciated. Or, conversely, the person may be afraid of *any* pain and have become so frightened at the possible experience of pain, that his or her very reactivity challenges the hospice team to maintain levels of palliation that the dying person can regard as adequate.

Because relationships and our understanding of them are crucial to providing excellent end-of-life care, a framework for understanding how relationships interact in a family system is essential for hospice professionals.

In this chapter, we will examine the family system theory first articulated by Murray Bowen (1978; Kerr & Bowen, 1988) and subse-quently developed by others (Carter & McGoldrick, 1989; Walsh, 1982). We have chosen Bowen because his approach lends itself to the interactions end-of-life care professionals have with the persons and families in their care. Further elaborating upon Bowen's theories, we will look at the possible meanings that a death in the family creates within the family system. Notably, in keeping with Bowen, very little of this discussion has to do with diagnosing individual psychopathologies. Our focus will be on the *functioning* of the system as a whole.

We start by examining the usefulness of Bowenian theory to end-of-life professionals. We then examine the conflict between a person's need for togetherness and individualism, and how that tension has an impact on family dynamics. We discuss Bowenian concepts such as emotional triangles, the importance of the family emotional process, and the multigenerational transmission process. We then show how genograms can be used to diagram the relationships within a family system. We end with a discussion of two other Bowenian concepts, the identified patient and societal emotional process.

This chapter is devoted to the dynamics of families in general. In the next chapter, we will apply this perspective to families with histories of addiction.

FAMILY SYSTEMS: THE BENEFITS OF A BOWENIAN APPROACH

We present a Bowenian approach to family systems to demonstrate its utility and adaptability in end-of-life care. We are not, however, advocating that end-of-life care professionals see themselves as quasi-therapists. In fact, it is to downplay the diagnostic and therapeutic aspects of most psychological theories that we have chosen Bowen's approach. Philosophically, Bowen had confidence in the inherent ability people have to change and grow if only they could examine and understand their family's behavior and dynamics in a more objective way (Kerr & Bowen, 1988). Bowen thought that each of us has within ourselves a capacity, which we can enhance, to "think about communication from another in a way that is not influenced by [our] subjective feelings and emotional responses to that communication" (Kerr & Bowen, p. 67). Related to Bowen's approach, Minuchin and Fishman suggested that families are dynamic and are able to adapt; approaches to families need to be dynamic and adaptable (1981).

Bowenian family systems theory recommends itself for use by end-of-life professionals because Bowen and his followers saw themselves less as therapists (in the sense of diagnosing and healing the various psychopathologies in a family) than as coaches or consultants or even teachers who would maintain a focus on how the family members interacted and encourage their reflection on that interaction. That is, a Bowenian family systems approach focuses on emotional *process* rather than the *content* of the emotionality expressed. A Bowenian approach would enhance the hospice professional's ability to remain "in" the family system without being "of " it. This kind of "neutrality" is better achieved when an end-of-life care professional develops the ability to ask the family questions related to how they function, as a strategic alternative to providing answers based on assessments of their personalities (Kerr & Bowen, p. 284). In this way, end-of-life care professionals are better able to maintain their own objectivity, even as they teach family members to be more objective about their relationships with each other.

This approach fits well within hospice in particular because of the relative brevity of end-of-life care. A short length of stay does not mean that hospice professionals cannot have a significant and positive impact upon the functioning of the family during their time of transition and crisis at the end of life. Instead, it means that the goals of hospice professionals need to be modest and that their skills need to be exceptional.

Because a Bowenian approach affirms the ability of families to learn more about themselves, and because the advent of a terminal prognosis for one of its members occasions a series of learning opportunities for the rest of the family, a Bowenian approach seems appropriately useful for hospice professionals. Just as the doctors and nurses on the hospice team teach family members about disease process and pain abatement, so might the social workers and spiritual care providers discuss the family's emotional process.

Hospice professionals do not have to work on *changing* the family. The family is already changing. Instead, it is the role of the hospice professional to *observe* the impacts of the change on the family, and to be able to *optimize* those impacts for the sake of the family's health. The hospice professional does this by participating to some degree in the life of the family, and by being able to leave that family at the time of or soon after the family member's death. Given the limited time hospice professionals have with any given family, we think it is helpful for them to see themselves as *catalysts* for health and growth in families undergoing this transition. And, as in chemistry, catalysts precipitate out.

FAMILY SYSTEMS THEORY: TWO PRINCIPAL VARIABLES

The essential dynamics of a Bowenian approach can be grasped by understanding how its two principal variables or processes interact. Bowen called the first variable *differentiation of self*.

For Bowen, all persons are born with two competing and opposite instincts or impulses (Kerr & Bowen, 1988). On the one hand, we want to belong; we seek *togetherness*. On the other hand, we want to be our own person; we seek *individualism*. These conflicting forces are constantly at work within us; they are activated whenever we are in relationships, and we certainly experience them in our family life.

For Bowen, the balance we strike between these competing aims of togetherness and individualism can be gauged. Bowen called the degree to which we personally balance our need for togetherness and our quest for individualism, in favor of the latter, our *self-differentiation* (Bowen, 1978; Kerr & Bowen, 1988, p. 68). On a scale of 0 to 100, with 0 representing extreme togetherness and 100 representing extreme individualism, only the most thoroughly individualized people have high self-differentiation ratings. A disciple of Bowen's, Edwin Friedman (personal communication, April 8, 1994), once said that perhaps even Jesus or Buddha could be said to have achieved only a rating of, say, 70! Obviously, most of us have significantly lower levels of self-differentiation.

Bowen further theorized (Bowen, 1978) that families and other social systems exert a kind of pull upon us away from individualism and toward togetherness. Simply being in a relationship is likely to challenge our self-differentiation to some degree.

Families themselves, as systems, can be gauged by their level of differentiation. Bowen understood these dynamics to work in families such that each individual would have his or her own level of self-differentiation, and the tendency would be for everyone in the family to be pulled in the direction of the *least* differentiated of its members with the gravity-like tendency toward togetherness being just that strong in exerting its influence.

The second principal variable in the Bowenian family systems approach is *chronic anxiety* (Kerr & Bowen, 1988). All systems experience a certain level of chronic anxiety and manage it by endeavoring to maintain a balance or equilibrium. More highly differentiated families have more options or flexibility, and thus experience lower levels of chronic anxiety than less well-differentiated families.

Chronic anxiety and self-differentiation exist in inverse proportion to each other. Moreover, Bowen theorized, the capacity for any family to promote self-differentiation could be measured by the level of chronic anxiety in that family. Families that can tolerate (and even appreciate) each other's differences—and not be made anxious by them—can be said to be more differentiated, because the capacity for individualism is not seen as a threat to the family's togetherness. On the other hand, families in which the individualism of one member provokes higher levels of anxiety in others can be said to be less differentiated (Kerr & Bowen, 1988). This "fusion" or overdependence on others prevents individuals from pursuing their own interests and achievements (Walsh & Scheinkman, 1989).

Bowen distinguished between the chronic anxiety persistent in a relational system and the *acute* anxiety experienced at the time of specific events (Kerr & Bowen, 1988). Although chronic anxiety is present always as a response to what might be imagined or what might be possible, acute anxiety arises in response to what actually *is*. Families with higher levels of self-differentiation respond to specific threats with lower levels of emotional reactivity and restore their system's equilibrium more quickly. Because their emotional reactivity is higher, less well-differentiated families have a diminished capacity to adapt to stress. Families with lower levels of self-differentiation and higher levels of chronic anxiety have a more difficult time restoring equilibrium and managing the additional, acute anxiety. For this reason, they are more likely to become symptomatic (Kerr & Bowen, 1988).

The Cinnamon family's reaction to George's smoking is a simple illustration of these concepts. Amy expects her mother to do something to stop him; Wilma allows it out of a sense of her own helplessness. And George smokes, knowing that not only is it bad for his health, but also that it irritates Wilma and Amy. All three are caught up in a system with a relatively high level of chronic anxiety that has been heightened further by acute anxiety in response to George's terminal diagnosis. Their heightened levels of anxiety are likely to persist throughout the course of George's dying; only after his death, in the course of mourning, will the Cinnamons arrive at another level of equilibrium. And given their relatively lower levels of self-differentiation, the likelihood of their becoming symptomatic in the course of this process is higher. In order for the staff at Heart of Gold Hospice to provide them with the best possible care, it would help them to understand the extent of the threat to the Cinnamon's family system.

To summarize, togetherness and separateness compete *within* us, to challenge our levels of self-differentiation, as well as *between* us, to produce anxiety when we do not sense that we are together enough. Thus, from a family systems perspective, *a death of a family member is less of an individual's experience and more of an event in the family's history that is experienced by the whole family*. It is an episode of acute anxiety which adds to the chronic anxiety already present in the family, further challenging everyone's ability to maintain the equilibrium of the system.

On the other hand, and perhaps paradoxically, *an individual's dying is often the most explicit challenge and opportunity to be as self-differentiated as possible*; dying is the ultimate self-differentiating process for the one who dies. The gravitation-like pull to continue to belong to the family is challenged and even overcome by the individual's impending separation from the family system. The impulse toward "togetherness" abates. This explains the interesting phenomenon that, often, the least anxious person in a family with a loved one dying is the dying person.

FAMILY SYSTEMS: ADDITIONAL BOWENIAN CONCEPTS

Other Bowenian concepts can further help us understand some of the dynamics in end-of-life care. We will pay special attention to how *emotional triangles* function and why; the importance of the *family emotional process*; how the *multigenerational transmission process* works, including the creation of destructive emotional processes; and why individuals in families use *emotional cutoffs*. We will also discuss Bowen's (Kerr & Bowen, 1988) concept of the *identified patient* or the *symptomatic person*. (This is by no means a complete repertoire of Bowenian terminology; these are, however, the concepts that we think can be immediately employed by end-of-life professionals.)

We will also mention McGoldrick and colleagues' (McGoldrick, Anderson, & Walsh, 1989) concept of the *family life cycle*, which identifies the variety of developmental stages experienced by families to frame their work within our focus on end-of-life care.

Emotional Triangles

Commonly, we think of relationships as occurring between two people. Thus our tendency is to think of relationships as *dyadic*. But Bowen found that it was better to explain emotional dynamics in terms of *triangles* (Bowen, 1978). Members of families are not simply in relationships with each other, but also with all of the others in the family. These relationships can better be described and mapped as triangles. Triangles may also illustrate the competing demands among and between others (Walsh & Scheinkman, 1989), as we will further illustrate in chapter 8, when we discuss team functioning.

Bowen theorized that the anxiety produced in the conflict between togetherness and individualism could best be managed if it was shared among all members of the family. By sharing the anxiety, a family could find stability. And the smallest, most stable relationship unit happens to be, structurally speaking, the triangle. According to Kerr and Bowen (1988), "Triangles are simply a fact of nature. To observe them requires that one stand back and watch the process unfold" (p. 134).

Second, families, indeed all systems, try to preserve stability. Bowen and others called this pursuit of stability or equilibrium *homeostasis* (Bertalanffy, 1969; Bowen, 1978). Homeostasis is understood to be a dynamic process. That is, the stability of a family or a system is fluid; anxiety may flow throughout the family members.

Triangles not only symbolize this homeostasis, they describe the pathways of the anxiety through the family, the interrelationships and alliances that are formed, in order to share the anxiety and achieve stability. This is a constant and ongoing process because of the dynamic nature of life: change is always occurring, and change threatens the homeostasis or stability of a family or a system's functions.

In the example of the resumption of George's smoking, we can see how the triangle among George, Wilma, and Amy functions by noticing how Amy attempts to exert emotional pressure on Wilma to alter George's behavior. This dynamic is what is behind Amy's previous decisions not to bring her children to see their grandparents as often as Wilma wanted; Amy had told her mother that she did not wish to subject her children to George's second-hand smoke. Withholding visits was another way Amy attempted to exert emotional pressure on Wilma.

But now, George's terminal prognosis has brought the threat of change to the family's functioning. The emotional pressure Amy puts on her mother now not only expresses the nature of the family's present homeostasis, but also the acute threat to that homeostasis that George's imminent death presents. We can hear the anxiety in Amy's way of speaking to her mother, and we can see it in Wilma's resigned response.

Family Emotional Process

Bowen's formulation of emotional process (Kerr & Bowen, 1988) has essentially three components: how our *feelings* and our *thinking* become manifest in our *behaviors*. All three are a crucial part of a family's emotional process. How we think about ourselves and others is related to how we feel about ourselves and others, and consequently how we behave, whether we are alone or with others. Moreover, it is often our behavior that reveals what we are feeling and thinking.

In therapeutic sessions with families, Bowen would try to elicit how family members *thought* about themselves, each other, and their situation. He emphasized thinking over feelings or behaviors in an effort both to support the family members' self-differentiation and to dampen their *emotional reactivity*—their responding without thinking about their feelings (Kerr & Bowen, 1988). *Reactivity* in a family system is an expression of its chronic anxiety and arises from the interrelatedness of its participants. Family members are less able to be objective to the degree that they are intertwined. This "fusion" not only affects their feelings and behavior, but also how they think about themselves and each other. Family members can become quite adept at rationalizing their reactivity. Their rationalizations have the paradoxical effect of reinforcing their interconnectivity. That is, their thinking itself becomes evidence of the lack of differentiation in the family system and the higher level of chronic anxiety its members experience. Bowen's strategy was not to modify behaviors, nor to elicit feelings, but to promote members' ability to reflect about themselves, their communication, and their experience of each other. Bowen's premise was that not only would the family's self-differentiation improve, but also that their anxiety would decrease to the degree that family members could learn to *think* about their interactions. Simply put, they would calm down and be better able to manage stress.

This is especially relevant for end-of-life care professionals, who serve families who not only have their own levels of chronic anxiety, but also are likely to be experiencing acute anxiety over the terminal diagnosis. In families facing death, four distinct areas of heightened emotional reactivity have been identified: disorganization due to the shock or denial; fear and anxiety related to the uncertainty of the future and the stress of caretaking; emotional lability; and a "closing off" or shifting to an inward focus (Rosen, 1991). Bowen's methods would guide hospice professionals in addressing these sources of acute anxiety constructively.

For example, a Bowenian professional might ask George, "Do you remember what you were *thinking* as you went to the porch to smoke a cigarette?" or ask Wilma or Amy, "Do you remember what you were *thinking* when you saw George smoking?" The Heart of Gold hospice staff using a Bowenian approach might reasonably expect that George, Wilma, or Amy, when responding to the questions, would identify an area of chronic or acute anxiety that they were feeling. This in turn would help the hospice staff better focus their care. It would also enlist the members of the Cinnamon family in their own care of each other. In this way, by de-emphasizing what they felt (*not* trying to identify with them), and how they behaved (*not* trying to change them), Bowen aimed to help family members to be observant about themselves and each other; to be more calm; and ultimately to be able to identify a range of behaviors from which they might choose, instead of repeatedly choosing one behavior by default.

As we have stated previously, hospice professionals are not expected to serve as therapists for any person or family under their care. However, they can benefit from Bowen's theory by interacting more productively with family members. Instead of inquiring about their feelings or attempting to alter their behaviors, focusing on their *thinking* can bring about positive results. By asking what the family members *think* about what is going on, hospice professionals can make themselves somewhat immune to the family's anxiety—and thus avoid becoming inappropriately involved in the family's emotional process. (The risks of becoming inappropriately involved in the family's emotional process will be discussed in chapter 8.)

The optimum role of the end-of-life care professional is to be a *non-anxious presence* for the family experiencing an imminent death. It is important, then, for hospice professionals to monitor the degree to which they may catch the contagion of the family's anxiety. By prompting the family members to *think* about what is occurring in their family, hospice professionals also maintain their own level of calm, even as they stay in touch with and participate in the life of the family. (We will also elaborate further on this in chapter 8.)

Family Emotional Inheritance

Bowen theorized that trends in emotional functioning within family members are inherited and predictable. He called this the *multigenerational quality of family emotional process* (Herz-Brown, 1991; McGoldrick & Carter, 1989). Stated simply: History tends to repeat itself.

The predictability of the patterns of emotional process within a family across generations is determined by a set number of ways that anxiety is handled in the system. Bowen (Kerr & Bowen, 1988), identified three:

1. conflict between the marital partners,
2. the overadaptation of one partner in an effort to preserve harmony, and
3. the focus of parental anxiety upon one or more of the children.

Each partner brings not only his/her own level of "anxiety versus self-differentiation" into the partnership, but also brings his/her family's emotional history. Then, as *external* forces (events that happen to the family) and *internal* forces (efforts to remain self-differentiated) affect the family's emotional process, the choices they make to handle the anxiety typically amount to repeating the same options they have learned from their respective families. This is how family emotional process becomes multigenerational and repetitive. Either the parents will choose to be in conflict, or one parent will accommodate the other, or their focus will be turned upon the children, or some combination thereof.

In other words, because of the limited number of ways anxiety can be handled in any given family system, and because the younger generation is taught the choices of the previous one, whatever patterns are established in one generation are likely to be passed on to future ones.

When George insists, against the interests of his health, upon a cigarette, and Wilma accommodates him, we can see the way they are choosing to handle chronic anxiety. We can also surmise that they might have learned this behavior from their own families of origin. We can see that Amy does not view this choice as beneficial. In reaction to her parents' actions, Amy may make another choice with her husband, or she might let *her* children know that *they* have choices by saying out loud something like, "I hope I never end up like my mother."

It is this inherited quality of a family's emotional process which end-of-life professionals often encounter, since it results in an apparent intractability or inflexibility on the part of the family under care. Yet, it is precisely this inherited pattern of relating that family members regard as "normal." In fact, if we understand family emotional process correctly, *no* family is truly "dysfunctional," but rather functions in ways appropriate to its own understanding.

Managing Family Emotional Processes: Closeness and Distance

Altough all family processes are understandable, not all are constructive. That is, not all family emotional processes promote self-differentiation within the system. As was mentioned earlier, the level of self-differentiation among family members is a measure of a family's health. Self-differentiation applies to both the ability to be one's own person and to stay in touch, comfortably, with others. How a person arrives at the balance of comfort with oneself and comfort with another is an indicator of that person's health. Families (all systems, actually) function in ways that either promote or discourage their members' individuality in favor of their togetherness or belonging. Because families (as in all systems) function by maintaining a homeostatic balance that manages the chronic anxiety shared by all of its members (participants), the range of choices or options that families/systems provide for their members to reach their own level of comfort with self and belonging distinguishes one family/system from another.

Basically, these choices are arrayed in two directions. On the one hand, some choices can be described in terms of their closeness or attachment. For these choices, Bowen used the term, relationship *binds* (Kerr & Bowen, 1988, p. 119). Each bind reflects how the chronic anxiety in the family system has been "bound" in relationships or attachments.

Although "relationships are by far the most effective anxiety binders" (Kerr & Bowen, 1988, p. 119), one result of these attachments can be a higher degree of reactivity in the family/system, especially among less well-differentiated members. One could say that the more the family/system values closeness, the more likely its members will be more reactive to each other.

Another range of options for binding anxiety in families/systems includes the family's degree of involvement with drugs, substances, and other self-destructive behaviors. The effects of these choices will be discussed in chapter 5. But here we want to note two things. First, that the *motivation* for pursuing these behaviors is the effort on the part of individuals to manage their experience of the chronic anxiety in the family/system. Families with higher degrees of self-differentiation generally manage their chronic anxiety without resorting to this range of choices. For one thing, the chronic anxiety in the family/system is experienced as less; for another, the degree of self-differentiation among the family members means that they are less likely to be emotionally reactive, both personally and to the system, and more likely to be comfortable with the way the chronic anxiety is bound among the familial relationships. Second, one can reasonably expect that choosing to bind the chronic anxiety in a family/system to behaviors comes about because the level of chronic anxiety is higher, the members of the family are less well differentiated, and thus their capacity for managing the chronic anxiety in the system simply among the relationships with other family members is diminished.

Thus, in addition to excessive drug and alcohol use, Bowen (Kerr & Bowen, 1988, p. 119) points out three other choices families offer for binding chronic anxiety within the system: The binding of anxiety to food, which brings about eating disorders (from overeating and obesity to anorexia and bulimia); the binding of anxiety to success (either over- or underachieving); and the binding of anxiety to physical health (either being obsessed with one's health or chronically ill). All of these are mentioned here because they relate to the variety of choices that have in common a sense of "attachment" or closeness.

Emotional Cutoffs

On the other hand, some choices can be described in terms of their "distance" or detachment. For these choices, Bowen used the term emotional *cutoff* to describe the ways individuals managed chronic anxiety by distancing themselves from the family system. The choice of an emotional cutoff is made in order to manage relationships *between* the generations. The greater the lack of differentiation or "fusion between the generations, the greater the likelihood the generations will cut off from one another" (Kerr & Bowen, 1988, p. 271). Some family members choose to remove themselves from the family in order to preserve, or gain, a sense of self-differentiation. Amy's remark about not wanting to be like her mother is an example of how a person in one generation might use an emotional cutoff as a way of (falsely) hoping to become better self-differentiated.

Bowen suggested that cutoffs signal the amount of unresolved anxiety present in any relationship—unresolved because the distancing results in only apparent resolution of the anxiety. The two most common forms of cutoffs are geographical/external (moving away from other family members) and internal (managing to establish distance through emotional withdrawal). Geographical distance is not in itself an indication of an emotional cutoff, for family members can stay in touch with one another and enjoy significant emotional support even if they live far apart. On the other hand, geographical proximity is not in itself an indication of a well-developed self-differentiation, since family members can emotionally distance themselves from each other.

What is an adequate guide in assessing a family and its members is the degree to which one can be objective about one's own family and the roles each person plays in its functioning (Kerr & Bowen, 1988). Key to this is a point of view that appreciates both who they are as persons and how they are together as family. Being more or less emotionally cut off from one's family is a matter of degree.

Amy's behavior is an example of someone who is attempting both a geographical (external) and an emotional (internal) cut off from her family, by living a certain distance away and being selective about when she visits her parents and under what circumstances. She would like to believe that she is better differentiated than her mother, but as soon as she returns to the family home, she displays a significant level of emotional reactivity. Unable to resolve her chronic anxiety internally by verbalizing her thoughts and feelings or by otherwise adjusting her behavior, she maintains a sense of herself as different and distinct from her parents (especially her mother) by keeping her distance, staying away, and keeping her children away.

We might begin to wonder, "Where is John in this family's emotional process?" As we will come to understand better in the next chapter, John has found it necessary for his own health and well-being to live even farther from his parents than his sister does. And for a period of his life, he used drugs and alcohol to manage his emotional process with his family. However, now that he has experienced a significant period of recovery, John is actually less emotionally cut off from his parents than Amy. We will come to understand this apparent contradiction better in the following chapter.

The Heart of Gold hospice staff might reasonably want to question John's behavior and assess: Is he better differentiated than the rest of his family? Or is he emotionally cut off? Bowen (Kerr & Bowen, 1988) proposed an assessment scale of 0–5 in order to quantify the level of emotional cutoff. The most highly cut off equals "5"; a person who becomes highly symptomatic when he/she is with other family members, "4," a person who is able to be in touch with at least some part of his family; and "0" would be someone who is not "cut off" at all, who, regardless of the geographical distance, feels responsible for and responsive to others in his family, and whom family members know they can count on (Kerr & Bowen, 1988, p. 325f).

For end-of-life care professionals, measurements of family cohesion and self-differentiation are only general predictors of behavior. They may help end-of-life professionals know what to expect of a family and the individual persons in it. But they should be open to receiving new information and revising their assessments accordingly. People are not constrained by these patterns, and there may be great variation in behaviors, especially at times of acute anxiety, which is precisely when hospice professionals enter people's lives.

It should be understood that chronic anxiety serves certain useful functions: To serve as a way of rigidifying the person's position relative to closeness or distance and as a way of relieving tension with respect to one relationship, even while creating it in another (Herz-Brown, 1991). In this way, chronic anxiety in itself, along with the individual responses to it of relational "binding" and emotional "cutoffs," is not to be judged as "bad." Bowen's terminology is meant to be descriptive of closeness and distance, of rigidity and flexibility, not to be judgmental of anything but the efficacy and the function of such arrangements. This is true both horizontally (among persons currently living), and vertically (through the history of the family).

The Identified Patient

When a couple or family seek medical or therapeutic attention, it is usually because one member of the family has become symptomatic; that is, their behavior or health has become such a concern to other members of the family that they decide to seek treatment. (Often, remarkably, it is not the symptomatic person that seeks therapy.)

In end-of-life care, it may seem obvious that the "identified patient" is the family member receiving hospice care. However, that is merely the medical point of view. From the point of view of the family, it may be the case that other family members play this role within the family. Comments might be made about the reliability or dependability of other family members, for instance. Or a family member may be incarcerated. Or there might be such an emotional cut-off that the "identified patient" is not even informed that the family member is dying. The role of "identified patient" carries certain historical implications which seemingly have nothing to do with the present terminal diagnosis. In their service of the family, all of these dynamics should be taken into account by end-of-life professionals.

THE GENOGRAM: MAPPING FAMILY SYSTEMS

Once the basic principles of family systems are understood, they can be mapped or depicted through the use of a family diagram known as the *genogram* developed by McGoldrick and Gerson (1985). Using certain standard signs, such as circles for females and squares for males, and then connecting them through one generation to the next, one can see patterns in the flow of the family's emotional process. These patterns are then used to interpret or enhance the understanding of the family. Although we model our genograms on those described by McGoldrick and Gerson, we will add to them an illustration of the particular needs of families at the end of life.

Returning to George and Wilma's family, if we use circles for Wilma and Amy, and squares for George and John, we can begin with a basic genogram of the two generations as seen in Figure 4.1.

We know that Wilma tends to accommodate George (certainly with regard to his smoking but perhaps in other ways as well) in order to keep peace in the family. In Figure 4.2, we depict this with three lines,

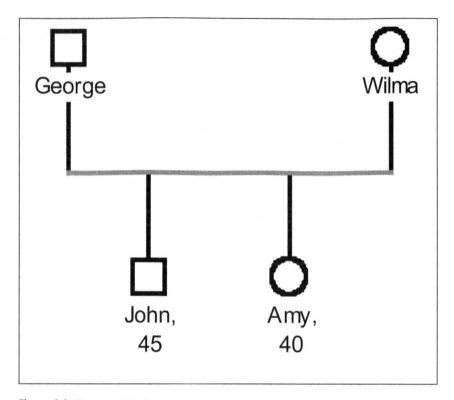

Figure 4.1 Cinnamon family genogram.

indicating a *fused relationship.* Moreover, we know that Wilma and her daughter have a closer relationship than John does with the rest of the family; we depict that by using a double line to connect Wilma to Amy, and a dashed line to connect John to the rest of the family.

Now, if we assess that John is, to some degree, cutoff from the rest of his family, we can indicate that with a slash across the line between him and his parents, presented in Figure 4.3. We leave a dotted line between him and his sister.

The advantage to using genograms for end-of-life professionals is that they present a great deal of information concisely and in visual form—conducive to the brief communication needed at team meetings. Moreover, genograms are flexible depictions of the family's emotional process. That is, they can be amended as more information is gathered.

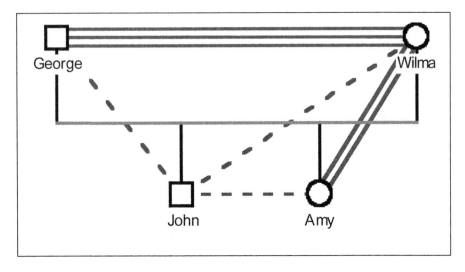

Figure 4.2 Cinnamon family relationships.

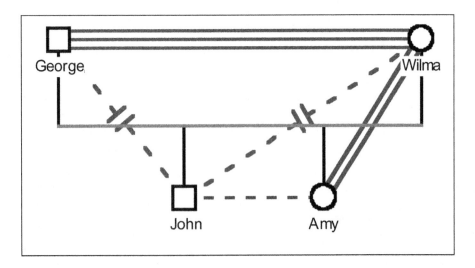

Figure 4.3 Emotional cutoffs.

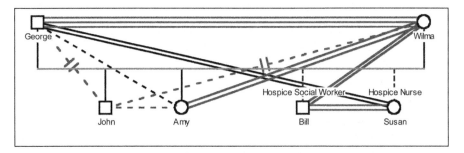

Figure 4.4 Heart of Gold hospice team and Cinnamon family relationships.

Thus they actually depict the team's deepening understanding of the family they are serving.

Genograms can also help end-of-life professionals to see who the family thinks *they* are, as they participate professionally in the family. In our fictional case, the two Hospice Team members might be perceived by George and Wilma as their idealized children; Bill and Susan get along well with the parents, but not as well with Amy and John. (The same aspects of a family's emotional process that might aid members of the hospice team in gaining acceptance from some family members might inhibit their acceptance by others.)

We can show this more effectively with the genogram in Figure 4.4. We have inserted Bill and Susan into the genogram, as if they are "adopted" children of George and Wilma (indicated with a dotted line). One might choose to illustrate them outside of the family genogram, but we insert them here because, in some ways, they have "replaced" the two children with their presence in the household, once hospice begins their service with the family. Note that we use double lines between Bill and Susan, as well as Wilma and Bill, to indicate the greater strength of those relationships.

The standard way to depict a death of a family member is to put an "X" through the sign representing that person. For instance, both George's and Wilma's parents are deceased, but George had a younger brother who died, and has a younger sister who is still living. And Wilma has two older sisters still living. Thus the generation of and before George's and Wilma's is depicted as seen in Figure 4.5, which reflects the multigenerational experience with death and other relationships.

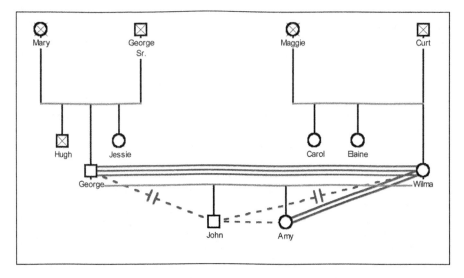

Figure 4.5 Multigenerational family genogram.

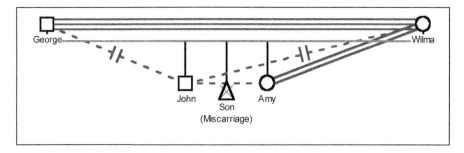

Figure 4.6 Significant life event: miscarriage.

Now, in addition to this information, the Heart of Gold hospice team discovers as care progresses that Wilma had a miscarriage about 2 years before Amy was born. We depict this event with a triangle, connected to the generational line, as in Figure 4.6.

Genograms are extremely flexible and can show all family events, including separations, divorces, remarriages, adoptions, foster children, abuse, health conditions, and a variety of emotional connections be-tween family members.

Within the genogram, no evaluation is made of any occurrences, whether they are good, bad, traumatic or beneficial—at least not without information from the individual family members about how *they* per-ceive these events. Instead, the genogram is meant, first, to produce an objective representation of the family's history, and to show the flow of its emotional process.

However, it may help end-of-life care professionals to understand the significance of deaths and other losses in the family's history if they think of each one in a particular way. In our experience, a death or loss in the family creates a kind of vacuum into which the family emotional process flows. As the family attempts to restore homeostasis, the closeness/distance configuration of the family is altered. This alter-ation can be depicted on the genogram.

For instance, the significance of Wilma's miscarriage to their family's emotional process could be depicted by drawing a line indicating "love" (a line which includes a circle) between the miscarried son and Wilma, George, and Amy. That loss created its own vacuum in the emotional process of the family, and had an effect on Wilma and George, and on Amy because she was the next child born. Being emotionally distant from the family, John was somewhat less affected by the event, so a dashed line (representing indifference) is drawn between him and the miscarried infant. This is illustrated in Figure 4.7.

A Point of Critique of Bowen: Societal Emotional Process

Societal emotional process is a term used by Kerr and Bowen (1988) to identify the sociocultural influences on family life. They acknowledged that society influences family functioning, but they took it to be a minor influence, and not directly relevant to family evaluation. However, two of Bowen's disciples, Monica McGoldrick and Betty Carter, argued that one could not fairly evaluate family emotional processes without taking into account the influences of both gender and ethnicity (McGoldrick, Pearce, & Giordano, 1982). Certainly, levels of self-differentiation in families cannot be adequately evaluated without taking the family's

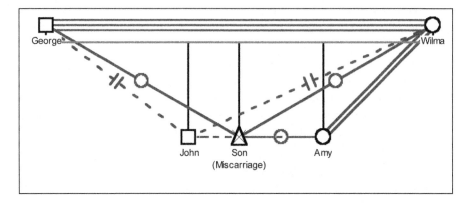

Figure 4.7 Grief and loss adjustments to family relationships.

culture into account, and understanding that the family's process does not exist in a vacuum. In fact, as a systemic approach to understanding families, it seems particularly important to consider those systems external to the family that impinge on its functioning.

Because families operate as systems, they strive to preserve a certain balance or homeostasis. In a parallel way, the internal tension between our individualism and our desire to belong has been said to mirror the disharmony between social needs and individual needs, as described by Ackerman (1958):

> [A]ll are agreed on the trend toward a sense of lostness, aloneness, confusion of personal identity, and a driven search for acceptance through conformity. One effect of this trend toward disorientation is to throw each person back on the family group for the restoration of a sense of belonging, security, dignity and worth. The family is called upon to make up to its individual members in affection and closeness for the anxiety and distress which is the result of failure to find a safe place in the wider world. (p. 219)

This description suggests that families are responding, in part, to external demands from the larger society (and its cultural aspects), and not just to tensions among and between their internal members.

For instance, Bowen's family system theories are particularly associated with dominant culture in their point of view, because they weight healthy self-differentiation on the side of individualism. However, other cultures place a greater emphasis on togetherness. Persons who are too distant or distinct are likely to be perceived not as healthier, but as more troubled.

Feminists also took issue with Bowen with respect to self-differentiation as a reflection of the gender bias that exists in the wider culture. From that perspective, there are larger contexts at work (social roles, dominance of men in families) that serve to influence mothers, in particular, to be "less differentiated."

This social critique of Bowen has suggested the need to be clear, when looking at families from a Bowenian perspective, that the lens through which he observed families was certainly influenced by the larger world and time in which he lived. Yet Bowen also made it clear that the goal of self-differentiation is to develop deeper relationships; thus, differentiation of self in relation to others, or being both separate and connected, *is* the goal (Walsh & Scheinkman, 1989). Although feminists correctly noticed Bowen's lack of attention to the role that culture and society played in shaping and even controlling the role that women in families fulfill, they recognized the importance of relationship and would likely agree with Bowen's goal of self-differentiation as *healthfully being in relationship*.

Knowledge of cultural differences becomes important as an "access" issue for hospice. As more people choose hospice as an end-of-life care option, hospice professionals will need to grow in their ability to assess families accurately across cultures. Hospice professionals would do well to assess this, and not expect all families' emotional processes to hold individualism in high regard. Bowen's family systems theory, therefore, is useful as a framework through which we might view the family, as it helps us move our attention from the individual to the family. It does not serve us as well in looking beyond the family to the larger systems without modifications.

SUMMARY: USING FAMILY SYSTEMS THEORY IN END-OF-LIFE CARE

To summarize this chapter, we offer a sample format of family systems concepts that hospice professionals can use to evaluate a person and family in hospice care.

There are some specific questions one might ask to gain an accurate picture of the family's emotional process, the levels of self-differentiation, and the effect that the terminal prognosis is having on the family system. Those questions include:

- Names, ages, and addresses of all family members, especially those in the generations immediately preceding and following that of the person with the terminal prognosis. (Aim for, at least, a three-generation genogram; however the more generations that can be included, the better.)
- Dates of marriages and divorces of all family members.
- Deaths, miscarriages, abortions, adoptions—whatever events in the family history contribute to an adequate and accurate assessment of the family.
- Levels of education of all family members.
- Emotional connections (both close and distant) between family members.

Once this information is gathered, then a genogram can be constructed that both compiles the information and gives an objective visualization of the family's system.

For instance, as the Heart of Gold hospice team comes to know George and Wilma's family, they learn:

- George is 68 years old, the second of three children; both of his parents are deceased; his older brother, Hugh, died 3 years ago, from complications of lung cancer, and his younger sister, Jessie, 66, suffers from emphysema; she lives in an adjoining state, in an assisted-living facility. George is the only one who married and had children.
- Wilma is 65 and has been married to George for 48 years; she had hoped they'd reach their 50th anniversary. She is the youngest of three daughters; both of her parents are deceased; she cared for her mother in their home until her death 2 years ago—just before George was first diagnosed. Both of her older siblings are still living: Carol is 68 and Elaine is 72. Both of her sisters' husbands died some time ago, Carol's in the war, and Elaine's in an industrial accident; neither has remarried. These two sisters moved in together; they live in the family's home town, three states away.

■ With George, Wilma had three pregnancies. The first and third went to term and resulted in John and Amy. The second miscarried when Wilma was 25. Wilma, who smoked when she and George met, quit after the miscarriage, blaming her smoking.

■ Amy is a 40-year-old mother of three children: Jennifer, 20; Brent, 17; and Gary, Jr., 15. She has been married to Gary, Sr., for 21 years. They met in college and are the only college-educated persons in the family, aside from Jennifer, who is currently a junior at a state school near their home. Amy began working outside the home 5 years ago, just before her grandmother became ill; but Amy's work prevented her from being as available to Wilma in the care of her grandmother as Wilma would have liked. Wilma thinks that a mother's place is in the home, and lets Amy know it. Amy argues that she didn't get her college degree just to "sit around and raise kids." Amy's husband, Gary, Sr., recently experienced the death of his mother. He and his sister (unnamed, younger) have grown closer since the death.

■ John is a 45-year-old divorced father of two, a girl, Serena, 23; and a boy, Johnny, age 19. He owns his own business—a roofing company. He and the mother of his children, Kate (44), were divorced when their children were young, and she was awarded custody, so he seldom sees them, but, Wilma says, that's only because of his busy work schedule. John lives in another town, 90 minutes away. His ex-wife, Kate, 44, and their children remained close to Wilma and George—closer, really, than to John.

On the basis of the above information, we can construct the following more complete genogram of George and Wilma's family, as seen in Figure 4.8.

Now that the hospice team has gathered this basic information about George and Wilma's family, what preliminary assessments might the team formulate? Among all of the family members, which ones might be better self-differentiated than others? On whom might the hospice team most rely in their care of George? What other observations might the team make? What other questions might the team members do well to be asking themselves, in order to be listening in an educated and anticipatory way for more information about the family's emotional process?

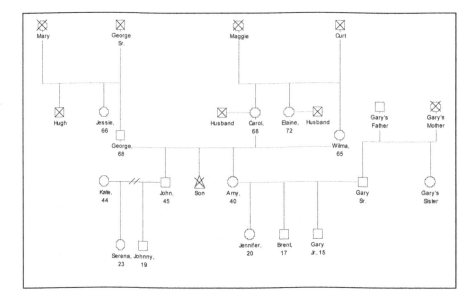

Figure 4.8 Multigenerational Cinnamon family genogram.

These are just some of the questions hospice teams might be asking themselves as they hone their care of families with members who are dying.

REFERENCES

Ackerman, N. (1958). *The psychodynamics of family life*. New York: Basic Books.

Bertalanffy, L. (1969). *General systems theory*. New York: George Braziller.

Bowen, M. (1978). *Family therapy in clinical practice*. New York: Aronson.

Carter, B., & McGoldrick, M. (1989). *The changing family life cycle: A framework for family therapy*. Boston: Allyn & Bacon.

Herz-Brown, F. (1991). *Reweaving the family tapestry*. New York: W. W. Norton.

Kerr, M., & Bowen, M. (1988). *Family evaluation: An approach based on Bowen theory*. New York: W. W. Norton.

McGoldrick, M., Anderson, C., & Walsh, F. (1989). *Women in families: A framework for family therapy*. New York: W. W. Norton.

McGoldrick, M., & Gerson, R. (1985). *Genograms in family assessment*. New York: W. W. Norton.

McGoldrick, M., Pierce, J., & Giordano, J. (1982). *Ethnicity and family therapy*. New York: Guilford Press.

Minuchin, S., & Fishman, H. (1981).   *Family therapy techniques.* Cambridge, MA: Harvard University Press.

Rosen, E. J. (1991). Families facing terminal illness. In F. Brown (Ed.), *Reweaving the family tapestry* (pp. 262–285). New York: W. W. Norton.

Walsh, F. (1982). *Normal family processes.* New York: Guilford Press.

Walsh, F., & Scheinkman, M. (1989). Hidden gender dimensions in models of family therapy. In M. McGoldrick, C. Anderson, & F. Walsh (Eds.), *Women in families: A framework for family therapy* (pp. 16–41). New York: W. W. Norton.

5

Applying Family Systems to the End-of-Life Care of Addicts and Their Families

Drinking at "happy hour" had become part of George and Wilma's routine from early in their marriage. For George, it was just a matter of living the way he'd seen his parents live. For Wilma, it was a change, since her parents only drank at social occasions. But Wilma thought being a good wife meant doing what George wanted to do. Besides, having George's favorite single malt Scotch ready for him meant that he would come home after work, instead of staying out at bars with people from his office.

As we discussed in chapter 4, Bowen's family systems theory suggests that humans have two conflicting desires: The desire for individuality, and the desire to belong. "Self-differentiation" is the measure of our individuality versus our belonging.

Bowen calls the tension between these conflicting forces *chronic anxiety*. This anxiety is experienced not only within an individual, but is also communicated in relationships with others. "Anxiety 'rubs off' on people; it is transmitted and absorbed without thinking" (Kerr & Bowen, 1988, p. 116). Family systems that both encourage individualization and tolerate the ensuing anxiety are said to be "better" differentiated. They are also relatively better able to manage the anxiety that arises in times of crisis or stress—what Bowen called *acute anxiety*.

Bowen suggested that the most effective way to *bind* or manage anxiety is through our relationships with others. However, anxiety can also be bound in our behaviors; for example, through the use and abuse of substances.

> Drugs are another binder of anxiety. Alcohol, tranquilizers, and illegal drugs can bind anxiety for an individual and within a family. The more the family can focus on alcohol as the problem, the more other potential problems are overlooked. Excessive alcohol use, of course, can also threaten a family and be a source of anxiety. (Kerr & Bowen, 1988, p. 119)

In this chapter we turn our attention to families with histories of addiction, using Bowen's position as our point of departure. It is worth noting that Bowen expressly names other means for binding anxiety: "overeating to the point of extreme obesity or bulimia or undereating to the point of severe anorexia" and "hoarding or overspending money and gambling" (Kerr & Bowen, 1988, pp. 119–120). We acknowledge that these (and other) behaviors may also be present as addictions. However, the focus of this book is specifically on addictions to drugs and alcohol.

FAMILY SYSTEMS AND THE PHENOMENON OF ADDICTION

Bowen wrote very little about the phenomenon of addiction, and what he did say was in reference to his description of family emotional process. In our observation, however, addiction as a means of binding anxiety functions in a distinctly different way. The reason for this lies in the addictive relationship itself. As Bowen describes it, the anxiety in the family arises within each individual and is transmitted, absorbed, and communicated among the other members of that system. As long as the anxiety remains an emotional process within and among other *persons*, the flow of the anxiety is dynamic; it can shift and move among the relationships each member of the family has with each other. That is, there is a fundamental *intersubjectivity* to the way Bowen describes *family emotional process* (FEP).

Addiction disrupts the intersubjectivity of FEP because addiction entails the binding of anxiety to an *object*. This qualitatively changes the emotional process of the family because it interrupts the "flow" of anxiety in their emotional process.

We have decided to define the emotional process of a family with a history of addiction as *addiction emotional process* (AEP). AEP is a variation of FEP that takes into account the consequences of having anxiety bound to an object. Throughout the rest of this chapter, we will discuss how AEP operates and the functions that it serves. Although our theories are based on Bowenian thinking, they are largely our own.

Addiction emotional process differs from FEP and has its own characteristics and consequences. This is because an object has no emotional process: It does not think, feel, or behave. It has no emotional reactivity. Although the object "receives" the anxiety being bound to it, it does not alter or process that anxiety; nor does it return the anxiety to the emotional process of the family.

In AEP, anxiety is bound to an object in an effort to stabilize the level of anxiety in the family system. The anxiety becomes "fixed" in the object, in an attempt to diminish the overall anxiety level in the family; however, this desired result is often not achieved.

There are several immediate consequences of the binding of anxiety to an object in addiction. When the family can focus on the *addiction* as the problem, other potential problems are overlooked (Kerr & Bowen, 1988, p. 119). Although addiction may serve as a distraction (and thus provide some immediate relief to the family's emotional process), it also creates problems of its own. Because "anxiety is an unpleasant but normal and functional affect that provides people with warning signs for perceived threats" (Marks, 1987), the family's reactions to other "threats" may be affected. That is, addiction is an ineffective effort to bind anxiety because it becomes its own source of anxiety.

The binding of anxiety to an object creates a shift among all of the relationships within the family. The manner in which participants in the system regard each other is also altered. A tendency arises to treat other people as if they, too, were objects, for control or manipulation, for example. When Schaeffer (1997) asks the question, "is it love or is it addiction?" and then proceeds to explicate the difference, she is explaining how addiction alters the nature of relationships among persons. Central to her explication is the role that *power* plays in addictive, as opposed to love, relationships. In addictive relationships, the attempt is made to manage one's own fears through controlling or manipulating other persons. This results in what Schaeffer calls "power plays." In contrast, in love relationships, power is realized within the individuals and shared in the effort to belong in healthy ways. According to Schaeffer, "in healthy belonging, partners work together to create an atmosphere of trust, respect, and safety that sets the stage for intimacy" (Schaeffer, p. 99). In our terms, in order for a healthy sense of belonging to be experienced, the intersubjectivity of the emotional process must be restored. From a systems perspective, this is essentially the goal of recovery from addiction emotional process.

FEP and AEP exist in an inverse relationship to each other. Systems that are less well differentiated have a higher likelihood of experiencing AEP, because their members are less likely to find other ways to bind the anxiety "subjectively" (that is, either intersubjectively through relationships or intrasubjectively through improved self-differentiation). But AEP and FEP are not mutually exclusive. On the one hand, addiction emotional process can be an aspect of *every* family's emotional process because the potential always exists for someone in the family to "choose" to bind anxiety to an object. On the other hand, even when AEP predominates, there still exist dimensions of FEP, because the possibility of anyone in the system becoming better self-differentiated is never eliminated.

UNDERSTANDING ADDICTION EMOTIONAL PROCESS

AEP becomes manifest in a family system when other options for managing the anxiety appear to be exhausted or ineffective. Circumstances that add acute anxiety to a family system already having trouble maintaining homeostasis can "trigger" AEP. By the same token, the family and/or any of its members can go through "recovery," which is essentially a process of managing anxiety by becoming better self-differentiated. These are not either/or choices. Rather, they demonstrate the dynamic nature of emotional processes available at any time.

How Addiction Emotional Process Works

Families with lower levels of self-differentiation have fewer options for binding anxiety. This leads to anxiety being bound through behaviors, addiction being one of the available choices. As mentioned earlier, rather than managing or diminishing anxiety in a family, addiction functions at best to *displace* the family's anxiety, by giving it an alternative focus. Ironically, this may actually *add* anxiety to the family system. In turn, this could lead to family members carrying higher levels of anxiety, and communicating it among themselves. When options for self-differentiation are less, there is a greater pull to what Bowen called the "togetherness force" (Kerr & Bowen, 1988, p. 121); yet this closeness or this belonging results in everyone in the family participating in a higher level of anxiety.

AEP originates when one or more persons in the family "chooses" to bind their anxiety (from whatever source) in whole or in part to an object, establishing *addiction* as the *family's* emotional process. Belonging to that family means participating in AEP, even if one is not actively an addict. AEP, like FEP, is characterized by a certain tension between the individual members of a family system and the system as a whole. On the one hand, the addicted person is attempting through the object-of-choice to stabilize his/her own anxiety. On the other hand, this behavior has consequences for the emotional process of the entire family.

When the addict binds his anxiety to the object, the object's lack of emotional responsiveness is experienced by the addict and the family as both *reliable* and *relieving*. In the family of the addict, binding anxiety in relationships has generally entailed a certain risk, because the responses of family members are variable. The nonresponsiveness of the object is thus experienced as being reliable. And the relief of not having to risk a response from a relationship, particularly one that might result in a higher level of anxiety, is appreciated (again, both by the addict and by others in the system).

The addictive binding of anxiety to an object can allay much of the addict's ambivalence about belonging. Because relief is experienced, the addict feels more comfortable about the relatively higher levels of anxiety experienced by belonging to less well-differentiated systems. The presence of the addictive object eases relational anxiety.

The addictive object does this both by contributing to the homeostatic stability of the familial relationships and by, as pointed out earlier, giving the family another focus besides its intersubjective relationships. The focus of the family's concern shifts from the *individual* to the *object*—it is the alcohol, not the alcoholic; the disease, not the person. Thus, the presence of the addictive object in the system provides both relational stability and a distraction.

Although the benefits of the addictive object attachment center on the stability achieved by "fixing" the chronic anxiety at a certain level, the difficulties with the addictive object attachment center on the fact that this now fixed level of differentiation in the family is relatively low. The results of this stabilized but lowered level of differentiation are chronic, and are reflected in the documented experiences named in chapters 2 and 3. The higher levels of violence, abuse, and discord experienced in families with addiction emotional process are indicative of lower levels of self-differentiation.

One result of AEP is that the family's emotions are drawn toward the one fixing its anxiety to the object. The addict becomes the identified patient of the family, the symptomatic one, the one who bears the symptoms of the family system's anxiety. The addict in effect relieves the family of having to process its excessive level of anxiety. The family arrives at its own sense of "normal." Whatever volatility is part of that "normal," it is at least predictable and thus familiar.

How Addiction Emotional Process Emerges

Addiction emotional process can best be assessed in terms of the *significance* of the object(s) to which anxiety is bound to the functioning of the individual and/or the family. We have observed that when AEP is manifested, the object(s) take priority over intersubjective, interpersonal relationships.

In our fictional case study, the Heart of Gold Hospice professionals would identify addiction emotional process in George and John because they are the family's "identified" addicts. But AEP has an impact on the entire family, and therefore signs of AEP are present in each family member. George and Wilma's history of alcohol use, and the centering of their life on happy hour, has had consequences in all of the relationships in their family. George, for example, has not established well-functioning relationships with his children. Wilma's relationship with George is less than optimal. Amy has made a habit of staying away from the family, and aims to shield her children from her parents, instead of encouraging that relationship. In other words, the Cinnamon's AEP might be identified in the impoverished and distanced relationships among family members, even in the absence of active substance abuse.

Hospice professionals who evaluate for AEP might take note of two aspects of a family's closeness. First, to what degree is it based on the use of alcohol or drugs? Second, they should consider Bowen's "togetherness force," which he describes in the following way:

> When people become more anxious, the togetherness pressure increases. During high anxiety periods, human beings strive for oneness through efforts to think and act alike. It is ironic that this striving for sameness increases the likelihood that a group will become fragmented into subgroups. We–they factions are a product of the pressure for oneness and the intolerance of differences associated with it. (Kerr & Bowen, 1988, p. 121)

In other words, when AEP is present, emotional closeness among people who are different from each other is not likely to be present. Instead, what is present is either a quality of sameness (we like each other because we are like each other) and a criticality of difference; or a sense of being oppositional, maintaining a persistent edge to the relationship in order to gain the appearance of distance, rather than distinct differentiation. When a family forms "subgroups," AEP is likely being manifested. In AEP the paradox is clear: Striving for sameness increases the likelihood of fragmentation; the pressure for onenes and intolerance of difference engenders factions and fractiousness. Thus, in AEP, the togetherness force substitutes for true intimacy, and emotional distance for genuine self-differentiation.

The Role of Shame as a Consequence of Addiction Emotional Process

The emergence of AEP has the primary consequence of bringing *shame* to the forefront of the family's emotional process; shame becomes more prominent than the anxiety already present in the system. Shame is not merely a common human experience; it is a universal one. Although shame is usually thought of as a "negative emotion" (Whitehead & Whitehead, 1995), shame also serves roles that are both safeguarding and constructive. (We will discuss shame more specifically in chapter 10.) Here we simply introduce that discussion by saying that once AEP becomes the predominant means for binding anxiety in a family, the principal consequence is that, along with anxiety, shame needs to be accounted for—"bound," in Bowen's terms—not just by an individual, but by the family system itself.

In FEP, anxiety characterizes the family's thinking, feeling, and behavior. In AEP, shame characterizes the family's thinking, feeling, and behavior. *The result is shame-based thinking, shame-centered feeling, and shame-management behavior.* The predominance of shame as an emotion that needs to be bound is what separates AEP from FEP. This does not mean that shame is absent when AEP is not manifest; shame is universal. However, AEP makes evident the presence of shame in the emotional process of the family.

From our family systems perspective, shame is the original emotion that gives rise to anxiety. Shame is "a feeling that one is inwardly defective, flawed, or invalid, and that one would be fundamentally unlovable to significant others if exposed" (Bricker, Young, & Flanagan, 1993). As all families attempt to achieve homeostasis, they grapple with both anxiety and shame. In particular, AEP serves to remind us of the importance of shame to the human condition, and thus to any system's emotional process.

Shame, blame, and guilt, often used interchangeably, are in fact distinct experiences that function in concert with each other, and occur in both AEP and in FEP—with the exception that AEP makes their interrelationship more apparent.

SHAME, BLAME, AND GUILT IN ADDICTION EMOTIONAL PROCESS

Because shame is a universal emotion, it is experienced by everyone and is an aspect of all families' and every systems' emotional processes. AEP makes evident the presence of shame in the emotional process of the family. This does not mean that shame is absent when AEP is not manifest. Even though shame in AEP functions in ways analogous to anxiety in FEP, the latter is not entirely devoid of shame to be bound, just as the former finds itself faced with binding both shame and anxiety. The anxiety of FEP does not simply evaporate or disappear because of the appearance of AEP. Rather, the continuing presence of unabated anxiety, bound and stabilized though it might have been in addiction, still weighs on the family and its participants. The weight of this anxiety is discovered in recovery, as those emerging from AEP strive to break the bonds of attachment to the object and become better differentiated. Whenever there is relationship, wherever there is a longing for belonging, AEP is present to some degree, submerged in those who are better self-differentiated, and emerged in those who are not.

Shame is inescapable for everyone. Just as Bowen distinguishes acute anxiety from chronic anxiety in FEP, *addiction emotional process is the experience of chronic shame, to which are added experiences of acute shame.* In FEP, only acute episodes of shame are experienced because the awareness of the family's chronic shame is diminished by the higher level of differentiation. This is why it is chronic shame that distinguishes AEP from FEP.

The function of chronic shame in addiction emotional process is parallel to the function of chronic anxiety in family emotional process. The shame of AEP must be "bound" within the functioning of the family system. Just as Bowen distinguishes acute anxiety from chronic anxiety, we can discuss the experience of chronic shame and acute shame.

There are principally three ways in which the chronic shame of AEP can be bound. First, it can be bound to actions or behaviors, real or imagined. This is how *blame* functions in AEP, to transform shame into guilt. Second, shame can be bound in the family's roles, rules, and relationships. Third, shame can be bound in the spiritual ways we discuss in chapter 10: in idolatry, isolation, and intimacy issues. All of these methods of binding chronic shame overlap, and function together in the sort of discordant harmony or volatile homeostasis that is characteristic of AEP.

Chronic shame cannot be bound in relationships in the same way that chronic anxiety is bound, because to a great degree, that option depends on participants in those relationships managing their emotions through self-differentiation. In AEP, that aim or hope has essentially been abandoned, in favor of stabilizing the anxiety by binding it to an object. The relational flexibility of the system (or among family members) in AEP is significantly decreased, and all of the relationships in the system tend to have become more static than dynamic, which can be observed in the existence of more rigid roles and the exercise of rules. In sum, chronic shame cannot be managed in the way that chronic anxiety can be in FEP because the relational option has already been abandoned by one or more of the participants in the system.

The Interaction of Shame, Blame, and Guilt

Shame and guilt are both "social" emotions that come from our longing to belong (Whitehead & Whitehead, 1995). Guilt is a consequence of our actions, of something we feel we have done wrong, an acknowledgment that we have failed. Shame is an experience of who we *are*, of a sense that something is wrong with us, or the feeling that we *are* a failure. Shame references our self-worth—or lack of such. "Shame is the name we give to the sense that we are unworthy and inadequate as human beings" (Bly, 1992, p. 147). Because shame has to do with our *being* as opposed to our *doing*, shame is, more than guilt, what participants in systems of addiction emotional process must "bind."

Blame and guilt become mechanisms through which shame can be bound in AEP. Blame is accusation, a behavior of assessment and finding fault. When a transgression occurs, blame is how the emotional process determines its meaning and the emotional consequence. It is blame that brings about guilt (either through one's blaming oneself, or through another's blame).

However, blame serves another function in emotional systems. Blame *transmutes* shame into guilt, by holding someone (either oneself or another) responsible for the shame one feels. In this way, blame transforms an experience of oneself into a consequence of someone's action.

Because families in AEP must bind chronic shame, they often use blame to change shame into guilt. The appeal of this process is that guilt would seem easier to live with because it means only having to face responsibility for a faulted action—not for being a faulty person. Yet one consequence of using blame to bind shame through guilt, is a higher incidence of blaming behavior within a family with AEP. Even when the blaming is shifted from persons to the recognition of the presence of addiction, the emotional significance of the blaming behavior does not decrease. This is because the prevalence of blaming is itself evidence of the need to bind shame, but the use of guilt constitutes an avoidance of the recognition that it is *shame* that needs to be bound, not guilt that needs to be passed around. Therefore, the binding of shame through blame to guilt masks the emotional impact and content of shame. When the family in AEP blames the object of addiction instead of the addict, or otherwise concentrates on the actions of addiction, they avoid addressing the shame manifested in the system by the presence of addiction.

The pervasive effects of shame can be seen in three ways: by understanding the stigma of addiction, by re-examining the psychosocial dimensions of addiction, and by understanding how shame is an aspect of the spiritual consequences of addiction.

The Stigma of Addiction in Addiction Emotional Process

Shame brings about strategies of *distance* among those experiencing AEP, largely because opportunities for self-differentiation are not available. In AEP the levels of individuation are low, and the immersion in belonging deep; as we saw earlier, this is one consequence of the "togetherness force." In order not to lose a sense of self completely, family members engage in other means of being distinct and different, instead of being differentiated. Those strategies are intended to "bind" the shame of AEP.

In AEP, shame first arises through the stigma of addiction itself. Shame is manifested initially when the addictive attachment is formed. When the *family* first experiences the shame-carrying consequence of AEP, it is because they recognize the addict is a member of their family; they bear the social stigma together. The identified addict may or may not experience the shame of being an addict, but the family does. It feels stigmatized by society, by other families, and, in turn, it stigmatizes the addict. All of this arises, not from *within*, as anxiety does, but from *without*, from the real or imagined regard of others.

To combat this, family members attempt to distance themselves from each other and the stigma itself. The stigma of addiction behaves like a social accusation—societal blame. Because the family cannot bear to be "faulty," it uses that blame to transmute its shame into guilt: Only the identified addict is guilty or at fault. In recovery (when it is a process undertaken by the entire family, not just by the identified addict) the family "takes back" the guilt that was the family's way of binding its shame. The family's claiming of its AEP as a shared experience is a step toward improving the family's health.

Anxiety, arising from within, challenges the emotional process of the family. But shame, brought forth by the regard of others, and thus arising from without, demands a different response: A response of hiding or denying. To bind the shame of AEP, families establish the roles, rules, and the sorts of relationships that they do. These become systemic strategies for dealing with the stigma of addiction.

The Psychosocial Consequences of Shame in Addiction Emotional Process

Family roles indicate two things. They indicate that family members have become defined not by becoming more themselves, but by the way they function within the family system. In this sense, roles indicate a higher degree of belonging. Roles also carry the sense of expectation: Family members expect each other to behave according to their role. This is how homeostasis is achieved. Furthermore, roles allow family members to distance themselves from each other because they do not know each other personally, as people, but only by virtue of the role they play in the family drama. Shame is bound to the roles in the family: Each family member knows his or her place, and if each person follows his or her role, shame will be lessened or controlled.

The typical *rules* of family systems (described in chapter 3) instruct family members what *not* to do: Don't tell, don't feel, and don't trust. Within AEP, these rules prescribe the means for family members to bind shame. Children growing up in AEP are especially sensitive to these rules, for instance, the need to keep secrets within the family. Secret-keeping is essentially an effort to bind chronic shame. As an Al-Anon member acknowledges, "Keeping secrets is common in most alcoholic households....These secrets only fueled our sense of shame" (Al-Anon, 2002, p. 59).

Finally, the *denial* among members of the family supports the family rules, and becomes one way for binding chronic shame. Denial is a refusal to see things as they are. Denial is ideal for binding shame. For if shame must be "covered," then denial is one way those in AEP can provide sufficient cognitive "cover" for themselves and for others. When the denial is adequate, then the family's homeostasis can be secure.

Denial works to bind shame not only conceptually, but also emotionally. "Shame suppressed does not stay silent. Instead shame recruits other emotions to speak for it" (Whitehead & Whitehead, 1995, p. 98); and two emotions that shame "recruits" are anger and fear. The levels of anger and fear in many families with AEP evidence the chronic shame being bound in the system. Denial displaces the emotional focus from addiction to, perhaps, something they feel they can do something about. By being a primary means for binding chronic shame, denial in effect expresses an acceptance of addiction and the emotional process consequent to it.

Denial as a means for binding chronic shame is especially important because families with AEP typically feature porous boundaries. Shame is a result of exposure. As Erik Erikson (1980) said, "Shame supposes that one is completely exposed and conscious of being looked at.... One is visible and not ready to be visible" (p. 135). The persistent experiences of intrusion, of feeling as if one is either constantly exposed or could be at any moment—all of the boundary violations are shame-producing. And they are common experiences of those in AEP.

In chapter 3, we mentioned the higher number and frequency of *losses* experienced by families with histories of addiction. In chapter 7 we will address issues of loss and shame more extensively; here we need only say that shame and loss are intimately intertwined. There is a stigma to loss in general; any loss will bring with it shame (along with other emotions, such as grief).

None of these psychosocial experiences leads to easy or constructive ways to bind shame. The surplus of shame at the psychosocial level functions to reinforce the addictive behavior. Addiction becomes its own way both of binding anxiety and of binding shame. This "double reinforcement" accounts for the rigidities experienced in addiction emotional process.

The Spiritual Consequences of Shame in Addiction Emotional Process

In addition, using the systems perspective of AEP, we can better understand the *spiritual* aspects of addiction. *Idolatry* is the spiritual term for the binding of anxiety to an object: The object of choice of addiction becomes supremely important to the addict, to the exclusion, or at least to the lesser prioritization, of all other (interpersonal) relationships. This in turn accounts for the *isolation* of those in AEP. The primary attachment to an object leads to the addicted individual being emotionally distanced from interpersonal relationships. We can now understand from a systems perspective why and how those in AEP experience *intimacy* issues. When one's primary attachment is to an object, then being in relationship with any degree of intimacy would entail a very challenging level of vulnerability. For those in AEP, intimacy becomes a matter of *control*, not closeness (Schaeffer, 1997).

On all of these accounts, shame arises: The shame of idolatry and object attachment; the shame of isolation, and feeling alone and disconnected; and the shame of being intimacy-impaired, so that, even as one wants to belong, the vulnerability and exposure required are more likely to bring expressions of fear or anger or both. Spiritually speaking, the management of chronic shame in AEP reinforces that process, exacerbating it and offering limited opportunities to escape or break the cycle.

It is because of the way shame functions in AEP that recovery is often envisioned as a spiritual quest or endeavor.

One of the biggest hurdles John faced whenever he began a process of recovery had to do with the word "God." He'd take the First Step, then in the Second Step, he'd hesitate. Even "God of his own understanding" did not help. Whenever he thought about "God," he thought about religion, and religion just seemed to blame him and shame him. He did a lot of work with his sponsor to come to a sense of what his Higher Power was, and to accept that the 12 Steps were spiritual, and not religious. What surprised him was, once he settled this within himself, he felt more comfortable about belonging—maybe for the first time in his life.

THE PARADOX OF THE ADDICT IN ADDICTION EMOTIONAL PROCESS

The functioning of the addict in AEP highlights the tension between the individual and the family system. A similar tension exists in FEP, and families can be distinguished by how they treat their individual family members and otherwise maintain homeostasis. A systems perspective on AEP explains how conflicting points of view about addiction arise; how the identified addict is regarded within the family system; why recovery is both promoted and resisted by the family system, and from this, the dilemmas that identified addicts face as they pursue recovery.

A Systems Understanding of Addiction Using Addiction Emotional Process

Up to this point, we have defined addiction as a subject–object relationship, explained how it stabilizes the chronic anxiety of FEP, and discussed the risks of chronic shame. Along the way, we spoke of addicts "choosing" addiction as a means of binding anxiety. By this, we do not imply that we support the moralistic and behavioral models of addiction. As discussed in chapter 2, the disease model best accounts for the persistently self-destructive "choices"/behavior of the addict.

The systems approach illuminates why we commonly come to this confusion: Is the addict responsible for her behavior and choices, or not? And if not, then is the addict being "driven" by a disease process as much out of one's control as, say, a diabetic's is by having diabetes? In the example of diabetes, there is an interaction of biological disposition and personal behavior. We believe our systems perspective helps understand this dynamic.

In family systems theory, whatever occurs in an individual is the result of that person's participation in their family system. There is no purely disease process that does not somehow express and interact with the FEP because the individual is never fully isolated from his/her familial relationships.

AEP functions in a parallel manner. Even if one sees addiction as a "symptom" manifesting in one person, the individual always belongs to a system greater than him/herself. When we say that a family member "chooses" to bind his/her anxiety to an object, we do not mean to imply that this is necessarily a conscious choice. It is not made apart from the family's emotional process, it is not exempt from the individual's desire to belong, and it is no more a pure act of the individual's will than, say, for example, "choosing" to be diabetic would be. That is, we recognize an *emotional process* at work here, just as significant as any disease process.

AEP is a *family* phenomenon, which may continue transgenerationally from one generation to the next, as levels of self-differentiation rise and fall within and across generations. What these describe, then, are *tendencies*—just as genes themselves are not always determinative, but in many cases indicative of tendencies. A systems approach to addiction takes into account both the individual's will, *and* that individual's participation in emotional processes with other people. Moreover, it is a more "organic" approach: it accounts, as physiology does, for addiction across generations. For these reasons we believe that a systems approach promotes a better comprehension of addiction.

The Regard of the Identified Addict

Understanding and appreciating the identified addict's participation in the family similarly benefits from the systems approach. It is within the functioning of the family that the particular paradoxes of addiction are evident. For instance, if you consider the addict to be "symptomatic," then you would expect the family to try to restore the addict and the family to health (the presymptomatic level of the homeostasis). However, in AEP, the opposite is more often the case. Instead of supporting the health or recovery of the addict, the family often isolates, disregards, or condemns the addict. Or, in an opposite manner, one might find that a family actually *supports* the addictive behavior of the addict. This is commonly called *enabling* or *codependency*. There is frequently at least a tacit recognition that the addict is contributing significantly to the homeostatic balance to the family—even when the addict's behavior is damaging to him/herself and others.

This range of responses within a family to its AEP displays the efforts of the system's participants to manage their chronic shame.

The Dynamics of Recovery

The family's tacit support can best be seen in the family's resistance to the recovery of the addict. For the addict, pursuing a process of recovery means detaching from the object of choice and becoming more self-differentiated. One would think that the family would support this. However, when the addict releases his/her primary attachment to the object of addictive choice, this releases the anxiety that had been bound back into the family system. Not surprisingly, all family members become more anxious—an emotional reaction made all the more severe by the lowered levels of self-differentiation among the family members. The "resistance" addicts often experience to their recovery from the members of their family, the skepticism they feel about their family's willingness to support their recovery, and the undermining of their recovery by their family that addicts often identify, all can be traced to the family's increased anxiety. The family is, again, facing the prospect of having to bind its anxiety in ways that do not promote addiction and its consequent emotional process.

In all systems, the change of one requires a change from all. In families with better differentiated emotional processes, such changes might be welcomed or regarded as surmountable challenges. But in families with AEP, changes are often viewed as threats. Embarking on recovery, an addict might find not only a lack of support but also that family members respond with accusation ("you want *me* to do what?") or a subtle pushback characteristic of resistance ("what will we serve if not champagne at the wedding?").

The family's emotional investment in the addiction of the identified addict corresponds to the system's feared consequences of recovery. For instance, Treadway (1989) noted that, "emotional reactivity is known to be more acute in alcoholic families" (p. 121). Given this higher degree of emotional reactivity, members are more likely to experience recovery as a threat. The threat is both systemic, that is, related to alterations and adaptations in the system, and personal. Because "normal" family life has revolved around the addiction of one or more of its members, other, nonaddicted members of the family may fear that, if the addict recovers, someone else will "have to" take that role, fulfill that function, for the family to continue to be "normal." Indeed, given the nature of the family, another member may become "symptomatic" in some way even as the initial identified addict seeks to alter his/her participation in the family's emotional process. This is one aspect of the insidious nature of AEP, and how addiction comes to be seen as a family disease.

This resistance to health and a healthy homeostasis is one of the hallmarks that separates addiction from other disease processes. Typically, families become more anxious when one of their members is ill; in addiction emotional process, families become more anxious when one of their members wants to be healthy.

This is also why families function better when each member in the family sees him/herself as requiring a process of recovery—not just the identified addict. In practice, this means that recovery for any family member, and thus for the whole family, can begin even before the identified addict embarks on recovery (and even in spite of whether the addict chooses recovery or not). Recovery is essentially a process of self-differentiation. Each family member can choose this option at any time, no matter how immersed in AEP the family might be.

USING GENOGRAMS IN FAMILIES WITH A HISTORY OF ADDICTION

We can use genograms to depict the alteration in FEP caused by AEP. In chapter 4, we showed how genograms could be used to illustrate basic family relationships and various emotional points within a family's

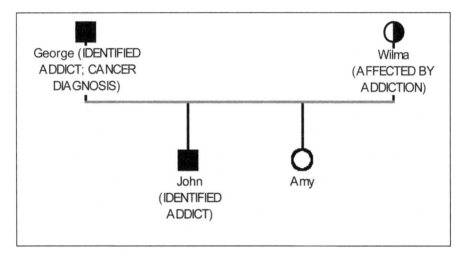

Figure 5.1 Cinnamon family and addiction.

experience. Now we will show how genograms can be used to illustrate addiction (in our fictional case study, we will start with George's alcoholism), and the family patterns that developed around it.

The members of the hospice team who come to care for George and his family will notice some things about the Cinnamon family right away, such as Wilma's request for privacy in the late afternoon (when she begins to drink) and the difficulty in meeting Amy and John, both of whom seem relatively uninvolved with their parents.

Once the team learns about George and Wilma's drinking habits, they might well begin to understand the effect that alcohol abuse has had on the family. They will want to represent this on the genogram in some way. We use a solid square to indicate that George and John are both identified addicts, and a half-filled circle to indicate that Wilma was affected by addiction, in Figure 5.1. We will also note George's cancer diagnosis.

We can take note of how George and Wilma's use of alcohol has established certain patterns of behavior between them, and between themselves and their children. This can be shown on the genogram with lines with an X—between all four members of their nuclear family, as seen in Figure 5.2.

Next, the hospice team would certainly find it relevant to ask about Amy and John, and their apparent noninvolvement. When they do,

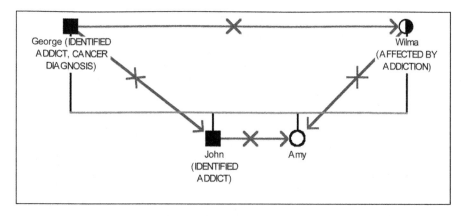

Figure 5.2 Addiction's function in the Cinnamon family.

Wilma discloses that John has had an alcohol and drug problem, that he has been in rehab, and that he has been sober for about 2 years—the span of time coinciding roughly with George's initial diagnosis of lung cancer. These facts can be included on the genogram by noting John's recovery, the onset of George's diagnosis, and by the double line that connects these events in Figure 5.3. Underscoring the latter two dates will highlight their significance.

The depiction of the Cinnamon family AEP allows us to speculate on some unspoken aspects of George and Wilma's family:

■ **There is a degree of isolation among George and Wilma and their siblings.** One might wonder whether this is due to geographical distance, or whether drinking (or other addictive behaviors) is present in their families. Some questions may help: Have either of them called their siblings to tell them of George's prognosis? What role (if any) have the siblings played in his life since the illness? Expressions of indifference or ambivalence *may* indicate a history of addictive behavior preceding George and Wilma's generation.

■ **A corresponding dynamic in the family's addiction emotional process should be apparent to the team.** George and Wilma might appear to the team to be a loving, emotionally close couple. But alcohol is what brought George and Wilma together; theirs is a pseudointimacy. In other words, George and Wilma's primary connection with each other is through their connection to alcohol.

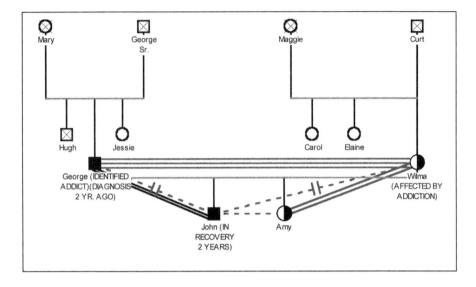

Figure 5.3 Addiction's impact on relationships.

■ **John's behavior could be especially significant.** His history with drugs and alcohol tells the team something about his level of self-differentiation, a capacity that is improving now that he is in recovery. Nevertheless, it could be regarded as tentative. The prospect of his father's death challenges him: Does he stay away while his father is dying and continue to gain in self-differentiation? Or does he risk those gains by re-immersing himself in the family's emotional process? Is the hospice team prepared, through their understanding of how addiction works, to help him make decisions that reinforce his self-differentiation? Or will they simply judge him as emotionally cut off, and not attempt to establish communication and support for *him* as his father dies?

The genogram can identify some of the dynamics present in the family, but cannot discern for us the answers to these questions.

UNDERSTANDING SHAME WHEN PROVIDING END-OF-LIFE CARE

To this point, we have described AEP in general and how it functions in the course of everyday life in families with histories of addiction.

From this general picture, end-of-life professionals can get some idea about what to expect when members of families with histories of addiction come to hospice care. They might better understand how the family has been functioning, and thus make more accurate assessments of their emotional process. For AEP is its own way of thinking about, feeling toward, and behaving in relationships with oneself and others.

The advent of a terminal prognosis for a member of a family in AEP is an announcement that the family is entering into a time in its life of acute shame, as well as acute anxiety. The family already experiences chronic anxiety in the course of its everyday life, and acute anxiety at times of crisis, as well as chronic shame. But in AEP, the anticipated and then actual death of a family member adds the experience of acute shame.

One source of acute shame is experienced through our bodies and their physical vulnerability, which becomes acute at times of illness, and all the more so at times when our vulnerability reveals our mortality. "Shame and death are close-linked," says Schneider (1997, p. 77) and he quotes Thomas Brown's *Religio Medici*, "I am not so much afraid of death, as ashamed thereof" (p. 81), written in 1635, to show that this is far from a contemporary sentiment.

This association of death and shame has become especially heightened as we increasingly rely upon medical technology to keep our bodies functioning. Schneider (1997) points out that we share a common confusion: " 'You do not have to die now' becomes blurred with 'You do not have to die' " (p. 87). Death becomes a failure or a defeat, both for medical personnel caring for the person and for the dying person him or herself. Either way, someone must be to blame for the defeat and/or the failure of the event of death.

The incongruity of death in highly technologized modern hospitals has provided some impetus to the contemporary hospice movement: From this incongruity has arisen the desire of some to die at home, in a more comfortable or familiar setting. The aim is to promote an awareness of how death is "natural."

The irony is that "sending people home to die," as their discharge from medical centers is often described, evokes shame. It transfers the shame of the failure of the medical situation from the institution (hospital, medical providers) to the family. The physician comes to be ashamed of her limitations; the patient becomes ashamed that he has not been a "successful" patient because he has not been "cured." And the family becomes ashamed that their member "failed" to get well; that perhaps they did not use the medical technology successfully and to its fullest extent—that they did not insist that "everything" be done; and that they perhaps did not do all they could. Thus, they, too, have failed.

For families who are already experiencing higher levels of chronic shame, the addition of acute shame may prompt a shame sensitivity or reactivity. When one is already steeped in chronic shame, one may be afraid of the possibility of feeling even more shame.

It is important for hospice professionals to realize that the referral to hospice of a member of a family with AEP means that the family's privacy has been breached—once more. The formerly "closed" family system has been opened. The family's defenses will be challenged. In some ways, the family's worst fears have been realized: They will be scrutinized and evaluated by *health* professionals. Families in AEP are already at least tacitly aware of themselves as "unhealthy." Now health professionals come into their home and acute shame results from this exposure, too.

The three ways in which this acute shame is manifest are congruent with the manifestations of chronic shame in AEP, as we discussed earlier in the chapter: through denial, boundaries, and losses.

Denial

Denial includes the attitudes and decisions that may have contributed to the terminal prognosis in the first place. The hospice team may witness a "perfect storm" of circumstances that arise from the use of denial to bind chronic shame:

■ Denial of the family member's physical condition may have contributed to that person's terminal diagnosis. Nearly all of the comorbidities that accompany chemical dependency, for example, benefit from early detection and treatment. Denial of symptoms and their significance may have contributed to the progression of the physical disease process.

■ Denial of the emotional impact of living in AEP can be one aspect of the chronic depression in such families. The prospect of another loss, a death in the family, and the anticipation of the changes to follow, with all of the unknowns that might entail, can overwhelm a family's denial and contribute to their stress response.

■ The "going public" aspect of switching from "private" medical care to hospice, which brings with it the fear (real or imagined) that "everyone" now knows that someone in their house is dying, means that the family's efforts to deny, to behave as if everything is "normal," will seem futile.

The acute shame of a family member's terminal prognosis threatens the AEP family's use of denial to bind shame in many ways.

Boundary Issues

One of the consequences of *home* hospice is that family members are expected to provide care for each other. The result of this expectation entails confronting *boundary* issues in any family, with the resultant shame (from exposure, body issues, gender issues, and generational issues). But in families in AEP, these boundary issues are not just matters of the present. These families have a history, which brings with it additional shame. We will speak about boundary issues and caregiving in families in AEP in chapter 6.

Loss

Finally, the advent of a terminal prognosis is in itself an anticipation of loss. In all families, this loss will have an impact. In families with AEP, this loss has additional meaning, for it is added to a likely series of losses that this family has already experienced. In chapter 7, we will address how the combination of chronic and acute shame affects the arc of mourning of families in AEP.

SUMMARY: APPLYING ADDICTION FAMILY PROCESS PRINCIPLES TO END-OF-LIFE CARE

The genogram presented in Figure 5.4 can help summarize what we understand of AEP and how we might be able to anticipate the challenges to caregiving for George within the context and history of his family. Figure 5.4 is a genogram of George and Wilma's family's addiction emotional process.

This genogram might remind us that we know very little about Amy, which suggests that we need to know more. Certainly the team's bereavement service is going to follow Wilma after George's death. But

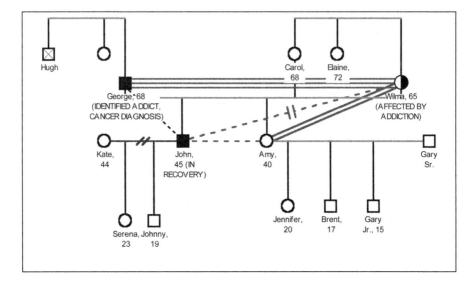

Figure 5.4 Addiction emotional process in the Cinnamon family.

the question might arise: Should Amy be followed as well? Or John? Or both?

The Heart of Gold hospice team can use the genogram and family systems theory to make at least a preliminary assessment. The team may predict that both Amy and John will be drawn closer to their mother after their father's death, because a death creates a vacuum, or an imbalance in a family's homeostasis. But because of the Cinnamon family's AEP, their functioning might not follow other families' patterns. For instance, John has staked his recovery on maintaining a certain distance from the family, so he is likely to resist the pull that George's death will create in his family's emotional process. This is likely to mean that Amy will develop even more of a closeness with her mother, one balanced by John's distance. The genogram can help "anticipate" this shift in the family's homeostasis.

The Heart of Gold hospice team might find themselves discussing some of the following questions:

> How *did* her parents' alcohol use affect Amy? How has it influenced her religious choices or spiritual points of view? What about Amy's husband—is there any history of addiction in his family?

How likely is it that Wilma will continue drinking after George has died? How will Wilma's relationships with her children change after George's death?

In what ways is the family likely to bind the anxiety released by his dying? How will the loss of his father test John's recovery? How will the closeness that Amy and Wilma forge following George's death be a reminder of the emotional distance John has experienced in his family? Anticipating these matters will greatly assist the tailoring of bereavement services for the Cinnamon family after George dies.

We now also understand that each of these alterations in the family's constellation will signify how it has re-bound its chronic shame. The acute shame of the dying and death of George will subside in time, as the family members mourn. We will understand this process better in chapter 7.

Meanwhile, the challenges of providing end-of-life care for families in AEP include managing both acute and chronic shame as the constellation of the family changes. In the next chapter we will see how a family's AEP shame management impinges on their end-of-life care. For the professionals of Heart of Gold Hospice, as for all hospice professionals, the reason they need to assess and appreciate addiction emotional process is to understand the nature of the caring that is already present in the family home when they arrived to start hospice care.

REFERENCES

Al-Anon. (2002). *Opening our hearts, transforming our losses* (p. 59). New York: Alcoholics Anonymous World Services.

Bly, R. (1992). *Iron John.* New York: HarperCollins.

Bricker, D., Young, J., & Flanagan, C. (1993). Schema focused cognitive therapy: A comprehensive framework for characterological problems. In K. T. Kuehlwein & H. Rosen (Eds.), *Cognitive therapies in action: Evolving innovative practice* (pp. 88–125). San Francisco: Jossey-Bass.

Erickson, E. (1980). *Identity and the life cycle.* New York: W. W. Norton.

Kerr, M., & Bowen, M. (1988). *Family evaluation: An approach based on Bowen theory.* New York: W. W. Norton.

Lee, R., & Wheeler, G. (2003). *The voice of shame.* Cambridge, MA: Gestalt Press.

Marks, I. M. (1987). *Fears, phobias, and rituals: Panic, anxiety, and their disorders.* New York: Oxford University Press.

Schaeffer, B. (1997). *Is it love or is it addiction?* Center City, MN: Hazelden.

Schneider, C. (1997). *Shame, exposure, and privacy.* New York: W. W. Norton.

Treadway, D. (1989). *The healing journey through addiction.* New York: John Wiley.

Whitehead, J., & Whitehead, E. (1995). *Shadows of the heart: A spirituality of the negative emotions.* New York: Crossroads.

6 The Challenges of Caring for the Dying: The Teamwork of Families and Hospice

George did not like what was happening to him. He had always been the sort of man who could take care of himself. But now, this was no longer the case. As he became physically weaker, he became miserable, because he felt like a child. He was short-tempered, and snapped at Wilma even when he knew that she was doing her best. He couldn't help himself.

Wilma, for her part, not only felt overwhelmed, but also angry. "He shouldn't speak to me that way!" she told herself. But she didn't tell George how she felt. She told herself it wasn't fair to him if she felt stressed, and felt as if she was caring for the most difficult baby in the world!

Caregiving presents its own challenges to every family—as well as to every person being cared for. Numerous demographic trends make caregiving more difficult now than ever before: Most notably, family members are increasingly likely to live at further geographical distances from each other. As the population ages and health care improves, people are living longer with more chronic conditions that require assistance. Yet, as modern families separate and relocate, there are fewer potential family caregivers living in proximity to those who need care.

Historically, families have been expected to care for each other in times of illness. This is true for end-of-life care as well. Hospices typically provide *supplemental* care; the hospice system presumes that the patient has caregivers available who will be able to provide (or pay for) adequate care. Yet the demographic trend toward distance in families (National Alliance for Caregiving [NAFC], 2004) has led to an increasing number of agencies that provide home care.

In this evolving social context, caregiving takes on increasingly important social and personal significance. In this chapter we will discuss the various systems of caregiving in our society, and the importance of caregiving to our general well-being; examine the paradoxical role that families in general play in supplying our caregiving needs; look at the special challenges in giving care faced by families with addiction emotional process; examine the role of hospices in providing end-of-life care; and examine how anticipatory grief functions, from a systems perspective, as family members begin to feel the transformation of their system as one of their members dies.

DIMENSIONS OF CONTEMPORARY CAREGIVING

Traditionally, there are three sources of care at the end of life: Through family (blood relationships); through one's spouse, partner, or friends; or through hire (paying others for care). End-of-life care often enlists a combination of all three. But increasingly, many different institutions provide care, either to support or to replace what has been traditionally provided by family or friends.

Caregiving Defined

The term *caregiver* refers to anyone who provides assistance to someone else. Anyone who needs ongoing assistance (medical or otherwise) with everyday tasks may receive care from someone else. Caregiving may be formal or informal and may occur in a number of settings. It may include care provided from a distance, or in close proximity.

Those who enter caring professions become "professional caregivers." Hospice team members are professional caregivers, as are those who work in home care agencies who provide services that hospice itself does not.

Thanks to advances in health care, more people are living longer with chronic and debilitating conditions that require additional care (Center on Aging Society, 2007). According to the Agency for Healthcare Research and Quality (AHRQ, 2004), nearly 10 million Americans need ongoing care, and 80% of that care is provided in the community rather than in an institutional setting. More than three quarters of those receiving care in the community get all of their care exclusively from *unpaid* family and friends (National Alliance for Caregiving [NAC], 2004). Their benevolence comes at quite a savings for the rest of us; the national economic value of unpaid caregiving is estimated at $350 billion annually (Basler, 2008).

In spite of the demographic trends which complicate it, the tendency persists to rely upon family and friends for caregiving at end of life. However, many people do not prepare for their end-of-life needs and the increasing dependency they entail, nor do they talk to their families about this (Bleiberg & Skufca, 2005). So it is not unusual that the prospect of providing care for George in his home, including the idea of involving hospice, may not have occurred to George and Wilma.

Providing private long-term care can be both physically and emotionally stressful. Because it is also financially costly (AHRQ, 2004), most people who need care depend exclusively on their family and friends; only 8% rely on formal care alone (NAC, 2004). In the United States, 44 million informal and family caregivers (or 16% of the population) provide care to adults over 50, according to the American Association of Retired Persons (Basler, 2008). Many of these family caregivers are themselves in poor health, and at risk for many symptoms associated with emotional stress (Navaie-Waliser, Spriggs, & Feldman, 2002; Yee & Schultz, 2000). According to the NAC, 41% of all caregivers are the adult child of the person needing care, and 22% of family caregivers are providing care for a spouse. Two thirds of these caregivers are employed at other, paying jobs. Many report having to take unpaid leave, rearrange work schedules, or decrease their hours in order to meet caregiving needs (NAC, 2004). Not all family caregivers live near their loved ones needing care. In fact, long-distance caregivers number close to 7 million (Wagner, 1997), and may travel 4–7 hours to visit the care recipient (NAC, 2004).

These statistics demonstrate that caregiving has an impact upon more than just the immediate family members needing or providing care. The needs for caregiving extend into the workplace and society at large. Moreover, the variety and types of caregiving relationships and situations suggest the necessity of a more comprehensive understanding of caregiver needs.

Hospice typically provides end-of-life care in people's homes (as they are doing for George). And they customarily support the family of the dying as they provide end-of-life care. This is why it is imperative for hospice teams to understand and be attentive to a family's dynamics, history, and to the delicate balance of roles, rules, and relationships in that family. It is just as important for hospice teams to provide adequately for the needs of those providing care as they do for those who are receiving hospice care.

Caregiver Needs

Family caregivers are considered a vulnerable and at-risk population. They often receive little support while performing exhausting tasks. For one thing, caregiving can be socially isolating, because caregivers often work alone, have little time for outside activities or friendships, and may need to quit working to meet caregiving's demands. For another, caregivers' risk for physical illness and mental health problems has been well documented (Goldstein et al., 2004; Shaw & Costanzo, 1997; Taylor, Kuchibhatla, Ostbye, Plassman, & Clipp, 2008; Tran, 2008; Zarit, 1980). Workplace absences and out-of-pocket expenses further contribute to the financial risks of caregiving.

Providing adequate support to caregivers requires a number of distinct areas of assessment (National Alliance for Family Caregiving, 2007). It is important for hospice teams to understand the following dimensions of caregiving:

1. the specific context for the caregiver;
2. the caregiver's own perception of the health and functional status of the one receiving the care;
3. the caregiver's values and preferences;
4. the caregiver's well-being;
5. the caregiver's skills, abilities, and knowledge-base for providing care (as well as their limitations in these areas); and
6. the potential resources available to the caregiver.

Initiatives to increase attention to caregiver needs have resulted in the development of increased resources to help caregivers and those who support them. For example, The Family Caregiver Alliance's National Center on Caregiving (www.caregiver.org) works to advance high quality programs for caregivers by providing extensive resources, including information about local funding and agencies, caregiver support, and help in navigating the complex systems of care that family caregivers must deal with. This organization has developed training manuals for professionals and family caregivers alike that acknowledge the complexities of caregiving, the need for support, and that coordinate the resources needed for caregivers who are often isolated and exhausted by the role of caregiving.

The National Alliance for Family Caregiving (NAFC) (www.caregiving.org), a nonprofit organization, has developed national programs designed to help improve services for caregivers and provide access to resources for caregiving. NAFC advocates for the importance of a consumer-driven, strengths-based perspective (National Alliance for Family Caregiving, 2007). This perspective takes into account the entire family system.

The Family Caregivers Alliance and the National Alliance for Family Caregiving are but two of many caregiver resources. However, it could be argued that, given the extent of the caregiver needs, these initiatives are as yet insufficient to meet the demand.

Caregiving and Hospice

Assuring that hospice patients receive the best care often depends on the alliances hospice professionals build with their patients' caregivers. Because caregivers have special needs and may need additional resources to do the "job" of caregiving, it is important for professionals to respect caregivers and the challenges they face, as opposed to assuming the role of "expert," thus undermining the family caregiver's role. This respectful attitude will allow hospice professionals to enter into the existing family system effectively and to supplement (rather than take over) the caregiver role.

Often the primary concern that hospice teams discuss with caregivers is patient safety. Although this is certainly important, interventions with caregivers ideally should also include support for their self-determination and self-care. It may also be helpful to teach caregivers a "self-management" approach, one that sees the family and family-caregivers as experts concerning their own situations. Professionals who work with family caregivers need to have good skills in communication and engagement, in addition to having knowledge of helpful resources to supplement care provided by families.

UNDERSTANDING CARE AND CAREGIVING AS RELATIONAL

We want to emphasize the point (as obvious as it might seem) that caregiving is about relationships. "The essential elements of caring are located in the *relation* between the one *caring* and the one *cared* for" (Noddings, 2003, p. 9, emphasis added). This is important on several levels.

First, when we talk about caregiving, we can envision a series of concentric circles: The individual being cared for at the center, the family at the first level of caregiving, perhaps friends at the next, and further circles related to programs or institutions of care for that person. Hospice, of course, is one of these; it functions in interaction with more intimate levels of care, such as friends and family.

As Noddings points out, how these circles of care function says something about how we function as a society. Her model for viewing care is an ethical one: The *value* society places on care, she says, underlies how we understand both care and caregiving (2003), *and* says something about who we are as social beings. Although caring certainly varies with both situational conditions and relational types, caregiving is rooted in our fundamental relatedness (Noddings, 2003). This concept of caregiving helps illustrate the importance of social support as an expression of care.

Second, caregiving itself is far from an abstract concept; it is a very personal experience of our common human *interdependence*. Caregiving itself is complex; it includes caring for, caring about, and being cared for. But its complexity is *inter*personal: How *do* we live out our experiences of being independent, dependent and *inter*dependent persons? Caregiving needs to include an *attitude* of caring, a sense of being accepted, supported, and loved. The caregiver's commitment to care demonstrates that the one cared for will not be abandoned (Noddings, 2003).

The relational necessity at the core of caregiving means that it cannot merely be a job. Caregiving may have its vocational aspects; we may value it—or undervalue it, as the case might be—in vocational terms, by measuring its economic and social impacts. But primarily, what we expect most from caregivers is that they *care*. Yet, what we least understand, perhaps, is that "caring" means different things to different people. Care has been called a "slippery and contested concept" (Brechin, Walmsley, Katz, & Peace, 1998), and at the very least has differing purposes, processes, and relationships that shape its complexities.

This is why caregiving comments both upon the nature of our society and upon the nature of our families. Caregiving among family members also highlights the ways they are independent, dependent and interdependent. This represents a key function in a family system's thinking: that each member or part of the system is inextricably linked to the other; any action by one person in the system has an impact on all persons in the system.

This leads to a third key aspect of caregiving: the interaction of the public and the private. We can certainly see this when we engage care from institutions and programs (the outer reaches of the concentric circles). We invite these public entities into our private lives (indeed, in the case of hospice and home health care, into our very homes), and we expect a certain quality of caring from them.

But even in the more intimate or immediate circles of caregiving there is an *exposure*, the crossing of private boundaries. Friends who provide care for other friends, and children who provide care for parents, are two examples of how caregiving entails the intrusion of the public into the private.

These encounters, or boundary crossings, often present challenges for both individuals and families. It may be difficult for some to display publicly what had always been private; namely, how the family cares for itself. So it is not just a matter of personal exposure or disclosure; it is also a matter of a family's *system* becoming known by those beyond the borders of the family.

How different families respond to these situations—how they know the care they are receiving is truly *caring*; how, or even whether, they rely on wider, social services for caregiving; and how they handle the matters of private and public interface that invariably arise in the course of caregiving—depends on the nature of the emotional process already functioning in that family. Next, we will compare and contrast family emotional process and addiction emotional process when it comes to caregiving.

CAREGIVING AND FAMILY SYSTEMS

There is no event quite like a terminal prognosis to test a family's system of caregiving. When a family member crosses the threshold into dying, how the family responds will reveal a great deal about how it functions to its members—and to others.

From our perspective, the emotional process of the family determines the family as a system of care. As we have discussed in chapters 4 and 5, *family emotional process* (FEP) is the way a family behaves to manage its anxiety during a time when its homeostasis is in transition. On the other hand, in *addiction emotional process* (AEP), not only is the family experiencing the anxiety of a homeostatic transition, but it is also concerned with the binding of shame. The role of anxiety and shame in caregiving, and the difference in their significance to a family's emotional process, has definite affects upon the course of caregiving. As discussed in chapter 5, for example, those experiencing AEP are likely to feel more highly exposed and thus more vulnerable while providing end-of-life care.

Caregiving occasions are times of self-assessment for families. Caregiving forces family members to ask: *What sort of family am I a part of? What kind of family do I belong to?* Most often, such questions are answered in terms of the responses of the individual family members to the need to provide caregiving.

The question of "what sort of family" is implicit in the assumptions people make about *who* will provide care when it is needed. The societal expectation is that family members will serve as primary caregivers. Even for those whose families are small or scattered, family, more than friends, tends to constitute the presumed community of care.

During the end of our lives, many if not most of us face challenges related to dependency. The independence and self-reliance to which we may have become accustomed—and that our society encourages—runs out or declines, and we may start to feel the limitations of interdependency within the systems of care we have constructed for ourselves. The question, "what sort of a family do I belong to?" takes on an existential urgency. It is no longer abstract. Very concrete tasks of personal care must be assigned to others. Those "others" become the "family" for those who are experiencing increasing dependence at the end of life.

At the same time, those who care for someone who is dying may find their own independence compromised. The dependence of the dying demands dependability from caregivers, and sometimes a caregiver must surrender his/her own independence for the sake of another.

In effect, there is a process of mutual assessment for both the one dying, and the ones providing care. This mutual assessment is never entirely objective: the family's emotional process will be tested by the caregiving that is needed and that which is provided—both by the family, and by professionals and volunteers.

This leads to our basic dichotomy between families without and families with histories of addiction—and to the possible contrasts in what "caregiving" means within each family system.

CAREGIVING AND FAMILY EMOTIONAL PROCESS

In a family without addiction, caregiving questions, as with all else, raise the challenge for self-differentiation (the tensions within the individual and the family for belonging versus individualization). How family members respond when end-of-life care upsets the homeostatic balance are expressions of their individual levels of differentiation, and the level of differentiation in the system itself.

The recognition that it is "*end*-of-life care" implies a period of transition. The previous homeostasis may be set aside, and a temporary one achieved. More likely, a series of temporary stabilities may be attempted and even maintained. In this way, the family system not only adapts, but also adjusts repeatedly in preparation for the changes that will come after the death.

This means that the world of the family is quite dynamic, even volatile, during the period of providing end-of-life care, and will likely remain so into the period of mourning. Some family members may be surprised to find themselves becoming more self-differentiated during this period. Others may become less self-differentiated, as they choose belonging to the family at the expense of their own individuality. Acts of caregiving nearly always require an adjustment in the direction of "belonging" in order for the family to continue to achieve a homeo-static balance.

We recognize this paradox: It takes a well-differentiated person to make a choice to "belong" to the family at the sacrifice of some of his or her own individuality. This is the paradox of caregiving: Caregiving most often occurs when the individuality of the one being cared for is supported and upheld by the one providing the caregiving, even if it requires the caregiver to surrender some of his or her own individuality. No wonder McCleod (1999) says that caregiving is "one of the most catalytic challenges any of us will face" (p. 13).

In family systems terms, the emotional process of the dying person is toward complete individuation as the pull of his belonging to the family diminishes. The efforts of others in the family to remain as differentiated as before actually works to increase the anxiety in the system, thus working against the effort to provide comforting, relaxed care to the dying person.

This is because the needs of the system have changed. The family that once might have supported independence now requires a higher degree of mutual dependence, and dependability. The ability of family caregivers to coordinate care among themselves is a mark of the system's interdependence, and of its members' comfort with the increased levels of belonging demanded by the circumstances. End-of-life care challenges the bases of self-differentiation in FEP because, generally speaking, it requires a higher valuing of dependence and interdependence.

We are not suggesting that persons providing end-of-life care should become completely undifferentiated in that process. But we are saying that caregiving, especially end-of-life caregiving, provides a unique opportunity for belonging—one that is both temporary and rewarding. To be able to adjust one's emotional process so that one can provide authentic caregiving to a dying family member, either individually or in concert with other family members, is the action of a well-differentiated person. This is the *benefit* of caregiving to the caregiver. Even when undertaken out of a sense of obligation or duty, there are opportunities in caregiving to continue the task of emotional development. Certainly, the benefits of this caregiving may not be realized until some time has passed. Nevertheless, many hospice caregivers will acknowledge, as research has documented, that caregiving has benefited the caregiver (Bellah, 1985; Grant & Nolan, 1993).

Caregiving for the dying often raises questions about capacity and limitation: How much can I give without completely losing myself? How do I care for myself and yet also care for my loved one? How can I both long for the person to linger, needing my care longer, and for him/her to die, thus ending the caregiving? Each end-of-life caregiver answers these questions, and others, for themselves. One can feel beneath such questions the anxiety imbedded in family systems. And in the answering of them, the alterations of family emotional process that all families experience after a loved one dies are accomplished.

CAREGIVING, CARETAKING, AND ADDICTION EMOTIONAL PROCESS

As discussed in chapter 5, families with histories of addiction must deal with both anxiety and shame. Those with AEP find the acute shame entailed in end-of-life care all the more challenging to bind.

In families with AEP the opportunity to provide care arises within a context of a history of *caretaking*. Caretaking, as we use the term, entails taking extraordinary responsibility for others, especially for the identified addict. In parents, caretaking is often evident in their blaming, either themselves (when they say things like "he wouldn't be an addict if it weren't for me...."), or others (when they say things like, "she wouldn't be an addict if her friends had not introduced her to drugs...."").

In children, caretaking most often begins as a survival strategy, an attempt to calm or control the family's situation by, for instance, trying to keep the alcoholic parent from drinking. As Al-Anon (2002) states, "If we were in the role of defending or protecting other family members, we may have an overdeveloped sense of responsibility for those around us" (p. 61). In many families caretaking begins as a survival strategy for the children of addicts. By the time they are adults, the role-reversal may have become habitual. The "adult child" may even speak matter-of-factly of having "always" been the "parent" of the parent. The difficulty caretakers face depends on the extent to which caretaking has become part of their identities, their sense of themselves. Caretaking is how they have come to know that they *belong* in their family (Wheeler, 2003).

Essentially, these are the functional differences between caregiving and caretaking:

■ Caregivers are better able to balance their care for themselves with their care of the one in need. Caretakers place the priority on caring for the *other* over caring for self, and resist having it any other way.

■ Caregivers *decide* to care; they have a sense of making a *choice* to care, and they make choices about how to care. Caretakers experience a kind of resignation: Choice does not enter into the matter, for they feel compelled to care.

■ Caregivers accept that they are to provide care as their loved one dies. Caretakers provide care while their loved one is dying, but they resist the reality of that dying; they are providing care in order to perpetuate the life of their loved one.

■ After the death of their loved one, caregivers are likely to ask: *Who will care for me, now that my loved one has died?* Caretakers are likely to experience a heightened fear of their loved one dying, expressed in this way: *If my loved one dies, who then will I care for?* Caretakers may be at an utter loss as to what to do with themselves afterwards, because caring for their loved one had become *the* purpose of their own living.

■ Caregiving is likely to end in a feeling of satisfaction, and an acceptance of the loss of the loved one, while caretaking is more likely to end in despair, or self-recrimination for not having kept the loved one alive even longer.

End-of-life care professionals may most easily identify caretaking (versus caregiving) through the confusion and denial of self-care. Family members may not know how to provide care to the one who is dying, *and* to care appropriately for themselves. Of course, to some degree, this is a universal challenge in caregiving, but it is especially prevalent and noticeable in families with AEP. In such families, the caretaker may exhibit a markedly diminished ability to define one's self separately from others. In fact, the *other* becomes more important, and in some ways more real, to one's own self.

Being unable to distinguish between self and other leads to an "all or nothing" approach to caring—"since I am caring for you, I do not have to care for me." The converse may also be experienced: "If I am caring for me, then I am not caring for you." This leads to fears of abandoning the other, of guilt over imagined neglect, and of shame for not "being there" when the other needed one most.

End-of-life professionals would do well to assess this moment in the life of those providing care. Is this an appropriate time for them to learn the difference between caretaking and caregiving? If so, then, the hospice team can encourage them to care for themselves as well as others. If not, then such encouragements are likely to go unheeded.

Her father's admission to hospice occasioned an almost immediate and overwhelming crisis for Amy. Didn't she have enough responsibilities taking care of her husband and her children? Hadn't she been paying enough attention to her mother and father already? In her mind, she'd been working to keep this sort of thing from happening. In her heart, she felt that her mother would never be able to give as good care to her father as she could.

This is what she was thinking and feeling, but she did not let on. Instead, she intensified her efforts to help her parents, and took others' comments about what a good daughter she was as encouragement to continue to do what she was doing. As her father's illness progressed, and she had to take a leave of absence from work, her employer appreciated the situation she was in, and her husband said that they could live on less for a while.

One of the difficulties of home hospice care is that it is only a supplemental, supportive service. There are occasions when a hospice team may find itself in *de facto* support of the caretaking being done. This may be true because the caretaker resists any attempts at self-differentiation. But it may also be true because the team finds it convenient to rely upon the family's method of providing care, even if that method involves caretaking rather than caregiving. Caretakers tend to be less demanding of hospice services. If the caretaking is not abusive, ineffective, or neglectful (which sometimes happens) then it may simply be more convenient for hospice teams to let well enough alone.

On the other hand, caretaking arrangements are sometimes more volatile; for instance, we have observed anecdotally that caretakers are more likely to call 911 instead of abiding with hospice guidelines. And caretaking nearly always results in complicated mourning (see definition in chapter 7), for the caretaker has not taken the transitioning time of the dying of their loved one to adjust emotionally to their passing. For all of these reasons, caretaking challenges the hospice team's provision of end-of-life care in ways that caregiving does not.

Caretaking and Dependence

The advent of a terminal prognosis brings a two-fold boundary challenge in families with AEP, both based on the likely violations of the rule of "*Don't Trust.*" On the one hand, when hospice comes, such families are likely to feel invaded. The boundary of the privacy of their family life being crossed, they are likely to feel defensive, wary of being scrutinized, and uncertain about how to handle the presence of the hospice professionals. Moreover, they are likely to be unsettled by their own dependence upon hospice to provide end-of-life care.

Families with AEP may have a higher stake in being perceived as loving and caring. Since they cannot completely trust their own assessments of their emotional processes, they are more likely to worry about how others perceive them. In other words, they need to *seem* as if they are caring, while at the same time they experience greater challenges to *being* caring, in part because they have learned not to trust each other. They are thus more uncertain about their ability to give care, whether the care they give will be well received, and whether they will actually receive the care they may need from each other. Questions of dependability arise—who is dependable for what, and, in what ways?

On the other hand, the activities of providing end-of-life care often necessitate boundary crossing. Boundaries are crossed in providing personal care or in simply witnessing the physical, psychological, and spiritual decline of a family member. In caregiving, these boundary shifts can be handled with courtesy and regard for the dignity of the one dying. But in caretaking, boundaries are already charged with histories of violations and permeability. Intimacy issues, active or dormant, are reopened and re-experienced in the context of providing end-of-life care.

As the dying person becomes increasingly dependent, the lesson of "don't trust" and its resultant suspicion engenders a wariness among family members. The tensions that are experienced by those who give care and those who receive care are often palpable and confusing. These are the hallmarks of a family in AEP endeavoring to bind acute shame when the means of binding chronic shame are no longer possible or appropriate.

Not only was Wilma reluctant to ask for help from Heart of Gold Hospice, but she also felt awkward about calling John. For one thing, he lived so far away. For another, he and his father had not been all that close. She couldn't remember when last they'd done anything together, just the two of them.

Wilma was thankful that she didn't have to ask Amy for help with George. Amy always offered! This eased Wilma's mind, that she didn't have to speak—her daughter seemed to know what she was thinking anyway.

In the course of their care, the hospice team would do well to replace any expectations of how the family *should* provide care with the acknowledgment that what they see in a family *is* how they express love. Affirming the family's caring is always important—and sometimes a challenge to hospice team members. However, it is not important that the hospice team assess or judge the quality of love expressed in the family, but only that the quality of care be adequate to the comfort and safety of the patient.

Caretaking and Independence

Another way in which boundaries are challenged concerns the ways family members *distance* themselves. In families with AEP, distance often substitutes for differentiation. Distance is one way that chronic shame is bound. The proximities demanded by end-of-life care challenge these distances.

End-of-life caregiving also challenges the rule of *"Don't Feel."* The impending death of a family member intensifies and focuses the family's feelings. Whatever balances in the emotional process had been tacitly in place become expressly apparent. This rise in the intensity of feeling in turn leads to an increase in family members' emotional reactivity. As these emotions are experienced, hospice teams often easily identify their relatedness to *grief* issues. However, what professionals may miss are the *shame* responses. Much of what they witness in terms of the fears and angers expressed in the end-of-life caretaking in families with AEP, stem from the efforts to bind shame, and the discomforts that arise because the levels of shame cannot be bound in their customary ways.

One afternoon, Amy found herself sitting in her father's room with him while he slept. She kept looking at her father, wondering: Was this the same man who raged at her as a child and frightened her so? Was this the same man who joked with her dates about the sex he was supposing they were having with her? Was this the same man whom she almost did not let walk her down the aisle because she feared that he would say or do something to embarrass her?

Yes, this was the same man. He looked harmless now, almost even innocent as he slept. But she remembered what he was like when he was drunk—and even sometimes when he wasn't. She hoped she would not have to change his diaper. Sitting with him, like this, seeing him, like this, was bad enough. But changing his diaper would be too much....

Caretaking and Interdependence

End-of-life caregiving also brings with it a requirement that the family coordinate care. For families with AEP, this challenges the rule of *"Don't Tell."*

During end-of-life care, everyone involved experiences a degree of interdependence that perhaps has not been experienced directly before. Not only does the one who is receiving care begin to rely on family members, but also begins to realize that in the past he or she had already relied on them, and likewise they relied on him. The ones who are giving care come to realize that they cannot do everything themselves, and they also need to depend on others. In the best of situations, a sense of teamwork develops among family members, and friends, and comes to include the hospice team.

However, in families with AEP, this required interaction challenges well-established family relationships, behaviors, and roles. How a family handles this shift depends on the family members' ability to communicate among themselves. Given the rule of *"Don't Tell,"* families with AEP are likely to be communication-impaired. Communication will be required with each other, with friends, and with members of the hospice team. The quality and quantity of the communication—what is said and to whom—reveals not only the patterns of communication within the family, but also the patterns of shame-binding.

We can understand this even more clearly if we remember the stake that caretakers have in providing care in families with AEP. The caretakers' sense of themselves not only affects their ability to bring order to a system that tends to be chaotic, but it also affects the ways in which they have bound their own shame—by staking their self-worth and their value as persons on being caretakers.

This means that caretakers themselves do not easily become "team" players. Theirs is a "closed" system—for reasons of chronic shame. With such persons, information is power. It is important for *them* to know, and also to control what others know. This is another manifestation of the secret-keeping common to families with AEP. But it also speaks to the significance of the patterns of communication in a family, and to why it may be difficult for hospice teams to establish a sense of interdependence and coordination of care in families with AEP. Each caretaker has a personal stake in being *the* caretaker. Shame-based family systems tend to perpetuate the notion that a failure to *do* something is because of one's failure to *be* something (Fossum & Mason, 1986).

As her father progressed toward death, Amy's emotional conflicts increased. Alternately she would feel privileged to be caring for him, worried that she was neglecting her own family, resentful of her mother for her failures to be a better caregiver, and confused as to what to tell her brother. Did John even know that their father slept as much as he did? She viewed the hospice care as woefully inadequate, but was afraid to say anything to them for fear that she'd offend them and that they would do even less. Hence she seldom talked to anyone from the Heart of Gold hospice team, but got all of her information from her mother. And since it wasn't much, she suspected that someone was holding something back from her, not giving her the whole story. She just couldn't decide whether it was hospice or her mother...

MEETING THE CHALLENGE OF CAREGIVING: HOSPICE AS A SYSTEM OF CARE

Hospice represents the interface of public and private systems within the concentric circles of caregiving described earlier in this chapter. It interacts with the family's caregiving system, but is an extension of external medical expertise. Perhaps no other part of our medical care delivery system depends as heavily upon having an adequate understanding of family systems and an ability to work with a diverse group of people (family members, friends), none of whom can be assumed to have medical training. In order for end-of-life care to function optimally; for the one who is dying to feel supported and cared for; for the caregivers to feel supported and cared for; and for the hospice team to feel accepted (if not appreciated)—it falls on the hospice team to understand the systemic aspects of this collaborative form of caregiving.

The challenge to doing this well is, of course, that not all families are the same. Hospice team members cannot merely replicate one successful effort over and over again. Instead they must constantly adapt their care to meet the differences of each family. Principally, these differences amount to this: Each family experiences being cared for differently. "Care" (or "love") is different in every family, and indeed differs among members of each family. One of the hospice team's first assessments is of *a particular* person's caregiving system. Hospice teams that are successful, adjust their own emotional processes to fit with the processes they find already at work in the family. We hope that by explaining the functioning of AEP we can further help hospice professionals be successful in their end-of-life care.

Hospice as Collaboration

When hospice teams collaborate with families in which the FEP is well differentiated, they will typically find that there is an inherent acceptance of and respect for the members of the hospice team. Their professional skills are invited, and their personal gifts are welcomed. Discussions about medical care are likely to be reasonable. Alternatives may be weighed and individual personal needs expressed without becoming personalized. Because there is a higher degree of self-differentiation, there is a greater ability to be reasonable and less likelihood of emotional reactivity, even through the stress of providing end-of-life care. In the end, hospice teams are more likely to feel successful in their caregiving with these families.

On the other hand, families with AEP will provide particular challenges to the hospice team. These issues have been alluded to throughout the chapter and will be summarized here.

■ Because family members have lived by the rule of "don't trust," they will experience problems with closeness. They may not be able to trust each other, or even themselves, to be caring. They might not even trust *caring* when it is shown for them. Hospice team members accustomed both to trusting and being trusted will find themselves challenged.

■ Because family members have lived by the rule of "don't feel," they are likely to have difficulties processing the intense feelings that can surface during end-of-life care. Hospice team members, skilled in helping people process their feelings, may become frustrated when so many feelings are processed so minimally or by so few.

■ These families may have well-established barriers to disclosure, and defensiveness about how they might be perceived by the hospice team. The likelihood of boundary violations, incidences of violence, chaos or abuse, or other matters of which the family and its members are ashamed, places challenges to the interdependence that must be developed if end-of-life care is to be optimal.

■ Resistance to change, or denying the need for change, may be more intense in these families. Shifting roles, necessary to the optimal provision of care, represent a threat or a risk in the family with AEP. Members of the hospice team may need to pay closer attention to supporting role transitions and to understanding the family's intense need to maintain balance and stability in ways familiar to them; distress and discomfort may persist even when, by the hospice team's estimation, they could have made changes that would have provided them with relief.

All of these aspects require hospice team members to be more flexible and adaptable as professionals providing care. During the dying of a family member, the entire family is transitioning, from familiar roles to those either less familiar or even unknown. The *functioning* of the family system is changing, which leads to both anxiety and shame.

The Hospice Team's Response

Because families with AEP possess a generalized suspicion about the public/private interface, and a guardedness about their family life, issues of control arise: Who do they have to "let in"? And whom can they "keep out"? Whose directions do they have to follow in providing care? Hospice teams can unwittingly find themselves in power struggles with the family over the care of their patient. These power struggles may mask themselves as issues of authority, when, from a systems point of view, they represent the family's uncertainties about what the roles and rules are in the changing environment of end-of-life care.

Because of this uncertainty, hospice team members are often assessed by family members on the basis of their function or necessity. Nurses, who provide medical care, may be seen as "good"—or at least required. Social workers and spiritual caregivers, who may inquire about the emotional life of the family, may be perceived as unnecessary or even hostile. Hospice professionals need to be alert to attempts to "split" the team, as family members identify some team members as "good" and others as "bad." It may also be challenging when family members select "favorites" within the team, and seem to exclude others from the sharing of information. Team members need to be prepared for some family members not to like or fully accept their help. Team members may not receive validation from these family members; they may need to rely on their own self-acknowledgment of a job well done, or feedback from team members.

Family members in AEP might respond to hospice in ways that are opposing or contradictory. They may both resent the intrusion that hospice represents and invite it. They may look to the team to take over care, and yet express anger at this possibility. Ironically, they may also express anger when the team *does not* take over care. In short, when the family has high levels of anxiety and shame, it will attempt to draw the hospice team into their difficulties, making it necessary for the hospice team to maintain appropriate boundaries, clear and direct communication, and non-judgmental, non-emotional assessment and intervention.

EMOTIONAL PAIN AND PALLIATION
IN END-OF-LIFE CARE

Not all of the dynamics just described will be evident in all families with AEP. What is likely to be evident is the degree to which family members are in pain. *Addiction emotional process* is painful. It is not just individual members who may experience this pain; the family as a system experiences this pain. Typically we use the term palliation to refer to the treatment of physical pains of an individual. Yet here, we will discuss palliation of emotional pain of the family. By recognizing that families in AEP are bearing higher levels of pain, the hospice team can attempt to palliate that pain throughout the system. The systemic pain may become evident in any or all of the ways we have described above, and sometimes erupts in violence and abuse.

In chapter 5, we discussed the higher instances of violence and abuse in families with histories of addiction (Barrett, 1986; Covington, 1982; McGoldrick, Anderson, & Walsh, 1989; Wilsnack & Beckman, 1984). These experiences present especially difficult and poignant dilemmas during end-of-life caregiving. If the one who is dying has been the abuser—who provides care for that person? If the one who is dying has been abused, should the abuser now be allowed to provide care? Hospice professionals may need to consult with experts on treatment of violence and abuse for specific guidance and enlist external resources to address such issues, and must be alert to the safety of both the ones providing care and of the one receiving it. The presence of an abuse history may indicate the need for more than one care provider to be present. Conscientious and more frequent and thorough attention to assessment of the provider's sense of strain or burden may be necessary. Hospice professionals may also need to be sensitive to the risks and benefits (to both the care provider and the one being cared for) in handling any confidential disclosures of information about past abuse.

The hospice assessment of patient safety must include an assessment of the safety of the environment in which the dying family member is receiving care, as well as the system that is providing that care. An assessment of the family as a *system* allows the hospice team to speak of safety issues directly with and among family members without appearing blaming, judgmental or alarmed (perhaps unduly). It is important that the hospice team, in raising appropriate safety concerns, do so in ways that not only address the pain in the family, but also mitigate the shame the family is experiencing. In fact, we would say that safety assurance, pain palliation, and shame mitigation are all goals that can only be reached adequately when they are reached together. In this regard, hospice teams should include in their pain assessments the physical, psychosocial, and spiritual aspects of pain.

ANTICIPATORY GRIEF AND BEREAVEMENT CARE

The anticipation that a family member will die also brings about the experience of emptiness—the anticipated emptiness that comes from contemplating, feeling, and even behaving as if the loved one has "departed." This process of anticipating the loss of the loved one and what life might be like afterwards is known as *anticipatory grief.* Anticipatory grief is an experience of the emotional processes *before* the loved one has actually died. Dimensions of this emotional process are indeed like grief, but since they precede the loss, they can be different in character and in kind.

The manner in which anticipatory grief is experienced is not in itself a predictor of the individual's mourning after the death (Rando, 1986). Factors related to the context of the relationship, however, do influence grief reactions (DeSpelder & Strickland, 2005). When construed from an individual perspective, the usual understanding of anticipatory grief focuses on personality factors related to grief. However, from a systems perspective, anticipatory grief and post-death mourning are different, each related to the constellation of the family system at the time.

Anticipatory grief, from a systems perspective, is the grief in which *everyone* in the family participates when one of the members of that family is dying—thus including that family member him/herself. Anticipatory grief is more than a personal phenomenon: It is the grief that the whole family experiences, as it makes the temporary adjustments necessitated by caregiving (or caretaking), and begins to anticipate the alterations that will occur in the family system after the death.

As in mourning of every kind, sometimes grief draws us together to comfort one another, and sometimes grief separates us into our own emotional processes. Sometimes those providing care to the dying provide comfort and consolation as part of that care. And sometimes, dying persons take it upon themselves to comfort and console those who are giving care, those who will survive and live on after.

In systems terms, anticipatory grief is an aspect of the family's response to changes in its homeostasis. The mourning of life as it was and the imagining of life as it might be is the contribution anticipatory grief makes to the family's emotional process. And the dying family member can very much influence the family's emotional process during and after the end of life. That is, the dying member can contribute to the manner in which a new homeostasis is achieved after his or her life has ended.

What tends to influence a family's experience of grief is the nature of the family's emotional process. If the family is able to balance togetherness and individualization, and thus maintain a homeostasis based on each person's level of self-differentiation, then the flow of the emotional process is likely to appear to members of that family, as well as to observers such as the hospice team, as "natural." That is, the family's emotional process will flow through and with the changes; adjustments will be made; continuities will be affirmed; and losses will be mourned.

However, in AEP, what the family experiences is likely to be a more tumultuous series of adjustments. Several aspects of AEP contribute to the emotionality in a family's anticipatory grief. Among these factors are:

■ The amount of unmourned and accumulated losses;
■ A sense of import of the moment, combined with a helplessness to make things better or even different;
■ The pervasiveness of denial, of pain, of the effect of traumatic events, even of the nature of the family's emotional process;
■ The fears that accompany shame;
■ The anxieties and apprehensions that accompany the invitation toward self-differentiation present during end-of-life care, regardless of the nature of a family's emotional process.

All of these may exacerbate the anticipatory grief that arises in the course of providing end-of-life care.

Hospice team members can best respond by remembering that what they are witnessing and called to provide care for is indeed a form of grief. As such, all of the emotions of grief are going to be present for all families during end-of-life care. It is not different in AEP. What *is* different are two facets or aspects of anticipatory grief in AEP: authenticity and intensity.

For instance, given the relatively higher degree of emotionality in AEP, one emotion that tends to get lost in the anticipatory grief of AEP is sadness—genuine sadness. Either the sadness can be replaced or obscured by other expressed emotions; or its perceived genuineness can be drowned by a flood of despondency. Given the conflicted nature of relationships in families with AEP, it may be difficult for members to identify honestly what and whom they are mourning. For example, how does one genuinely mourn the loss of a family member by whom one was abused or neglected?

The family's difficulties in determining what they *do* feel rather than what they *should* feel leads to their own acute shame. This acute shame is especially difficult to bind because of the cultural expectation itself of joining sadness to grief. When in AEP, a family's sadness seems either strained or exaggerated—what hospice team members are witnessing, from a systems point of view, is the family's efforts to bind the acute shame of anticipatory grief. (As we will see in chapter 7, this difficulty persists in mourning itself.)

In all families, the end of life is a reminder of previous losses and earlier grief. Thus, during anticipatory grief, it can be expected that memories, thoughts, feelings, and behaviors related to earlier times in a family's life will surface. This experience occurs regardless of the nature of emotional process of the family. But in families with AEP, these memories can bring resentment and anger at a more intense level than either the family or the hospice team might expect.

Resentment is a second facet to anticipatory grief in AEP. Resentment is the refeeling of past harms. Resentment contains tones of anger, sadness, frustration, even helplessness. In addition, there are elements of fear and apprehension in resentment. The result may be an increase in avoidant behaviors, short tempers, or brooding memories of things not accomplished. The emergence of "surplus" resentment in AEP at the end of life is essentially a *grief* issue. End-of-life professionals would do well to realize there is a history to these expressions of the addiction emotional process.

John didn't know why, but throughout the weeks his father was receiving Heart of Gold hospice care, he would experience these waves of emotion washing over him. Sometimes, he felt very sad, and would find himself weepy, seemingly for no reason. When he mentioned to Amy that he felt sad that their dad was dying, she responded in anger: "Of course, we're sad! What else are we supposed to feel?"

But when John talked to his sponsor about it, his sponsor told him two things. "John," he said, "you're mourning the dream. The dream that you grew up in a 'normal' household, or that you could be part of a 'normal' family—that's what's dying. Not just your dad." Hearing this, John burst into tears. His sponsor waited until John could listen, and then he said, "John, don't be surprised if you find yourself feeling really angry sometimes. It just comes with the territory. Work the Steps. Identify your resentments. Do what you need to do. You'll be fine."

SUMMARY

Caregiving at the end of someone's life is like giving them an extended embrace, even as they flow from one's arms. The period of time in which a family member dies (whether on hospice care or not) can be either a caldron or a crucible for that family's emotional process. If a caldron, then the family will merely "stew" in the juices of their emotional process. If a crucible, then the family will find that caring for a dying family member is an event that can positively transform their family and improve its emotional process. This is true for all families, even those experiencing AEP.

It thus becomes the role for the hospice team to supply guidelines for families in their care. As purveyors of realistic hope and guidance toward transformation, hospice teams can make a difference in every family's emotional process.

To do this, hospice teams should remember that families care for each other in many and varying ways. Sometimes the ways that families care for each other are either unfamiliar to hospice team members or make them uncomfortable. Thus it is important to be discerning about what each family defines "love" or "care" to be.

Second, the hospice team arrives in the family's life at a time when the family's homeostasis is in transition. Their familiar emotional process is in flux. What the hospice team observes and experiences is by no means the "normal" or "usual" life of this family, but is instead the family in crisis.

Third, families with AEP are especially vulnerable to the breach of private/public boundaries that accepting in-home hospice entails. Thus, they need both to be well understood and to be cared for compassionately.

In sum, the challenges of providing professional end-of-life caregiving to families with AEP include:

- To trust them, when they may not trust themselves;
- To speak with them, when they may not be speaking to each other; and
- To demonstrate appropriate levels of feeling and emotional responsiveness, when they may be unsure about what to feel, or even whether to feel at all.

Meeting these challenges, in whole or even in part, can be healing not only for the persons and families being cared for by the hospice team, but for individual team members as well.

The night George died, Wilma woke with a start and went to his bedside. George's breathing had become so shallow that she wasn't sure at first whether he even was still breathing. Wilma sat there, not quite knowing what to do. She wanted to turn off the light, but George had insisted it be on—back when he could insist on anything. She watched him, thought about their marriage, told herself to remember the happy times. She dozed, in spite of herself.

About 5 o'clock in the morning, she looked at George and knew immediately that something was different. His hands were very cold, his nails blue. Clearly, he was dead. Suddenly, she sank into her chair and began sobbing. She had forgotten to tell him "good-bye." She had even forgotten to tell him she loved him!

Later that morning Amy and then John arrived. They called the mortuary and hospice. John made some coffee, but every sound he made in the kitchen was like a hammer hitting glass. Why did the coffee pot have to be so loud? They sat for the longest while in silence, not quite knowing what to say to each other.

REFERENCES

Agency for Healthcare Research and Quality. (2004). *Long term care, Medicare costs, and use of hospice care.* Washington, DC: Author.

Al-Anon. (2002). *Opening our hearts, transforming our losses* (p. 59). New York: Alcoholics Anonymous World Services.

Basler, B. (2008, September 8). Care for the caregiver. *AARP bulletin today.* Washington, DC: AARP.

Bellah, R., Madsen, R., Sullivan, W., Swidler, A., & Topton, S. (1986). *Habits of the heart.* New York: Harper and Row.

Bleiberg, J., & Skufca, L. (2005). Clergy dual relationships, boundaries, and attachment. *Pastoral Psychology, 54*(1), 3–23.

Brechin, A., Walmsley, J., Katz, J., & Peace, S. (1998). *Care matters.* Thousand Oaks, CA: Sage.

Center on Aging Society. (2007). *Data profiles for family caregivers of older persons.* Washington, DC: Georgetown University. Retrieved June 1, 2007, from http: ihcrp. georgetown.edu/agingsociety/profiles

Cooper, M., & Lesser, J. (2002). *Clinical social work practice: An integrated approach.* Boston: Allyn & Bacon.

Corcoran, M., & Barrett, K. (1986). Family caregiving roles and burden. *Journal of Physical and Occupational Therapy in Geriatrics, 4*(3), 5–22.

Covington, S. (1982). Sex and violence: Unmentionables in alcoholism treatment. *Journal of Studies on Alcohol, 40*(1), 89–116.

DeSpelder, L., & Strickland, A. (2005). *The last dance: Encountering death and dying.* Boston: McGraw-Hill.

Fossum, M., & Mason, M. (1986). *Facing shame: Families in recovery.* New York: W. W. Norton.

Goldstein, N., Concato, J., Fried, T., Kasl, S., Johnson, R., & Bradley, E. (2004). Factors associated with caregiver burden among caregivers of terminally ill patients with cancer. *Journal of Palliative Care, 20*(1), 38–43.

Grant, G., & Nolan, M. (1993). Informal carers: Sources and concomitants of satisfaction. *Health and Social Care, 1,* 147–159.

McGoldrick, M., & Gerson, R. (1985). *Genograms in family assessment.* New York: W. W. Norton.

Navaie-Waliser, M., Spriggs, A., & Feldman, P. (2002). Informal caregiving: Differential experiences by gender. *Medical Care, 40*(12), 1249–1259.

National Alliance for Caregiving. (2004). *Caregiving in the U.S.* Washington, DC: Author.

National Alliance for Family Caregiving. (2007). *Resources for caregivers.* New York: Metropolitan Life Insurance Company. Retrieved March 7, 2007, from http: www.caregiving.org/pubs/brochures

Noddings, N. (2003). *Caring.* Berkeley, CA: University of California Press.

Rando, T. (1986). *Loss and anticipatory grief* (p. 24). Lexington, MA: Lexington Books.

Taylor, D., Kuchibhatla, M., Ostbye, T., Plassman, B., & Clipp, E. (2008). The effect of spousal caregiving and bereavement on depressive symptons. *Aging and Mental Health, 12*(1), 100–107.

Tran, M. (2008). Caregiving stress process: Examining the influence of transitions on caregiver health. *Disssertation Abstracts International, B, 68*(10-B), 6985.

Wagner, D. L. (1997). *A comparative analysis of caregiver data for caregivers of the elderly.* Washington, DC: National Alliance for Caregiving.

Wheeler, G. (2003). Shame, guilt, and codependency: Dana's world. In R. G. Lee & G. Wheeler (Eds.), *The voice of shame* (p. 203f). Cambridge, MA: Gestalt Press.

Yee, D., & Schultz, R. (2000). Recognizing diversity and moving toward cultural competence. *Generations, 26*(3), 6–10.

Zarit, S. (1980). Relatives of the impaired elderly: Correlates of feelings of burden. *The Gerontologist, 20*(6), 649–655.

Applying Family Systems to the Bereavement Care of Families With Addiction Emotional Process

Wilma stood alone in her home, staring out through the French doors. George had died a couple of weeks ago. The family and friends who had come to support her had now returned to their lives. It was that quiet part of the day, the part she and George had called "happy hour." Wilma poured herself a drink, as usual. But she did not drink it. Only after the sun set did she realize that time had passed. In the growing dark, she sat, holding her gaze on George's empty chair.

Grief is our human response to loss and is expressed with a complex constellation of feelings: Sadness, pain, worry and fear, anger or frustration, and confusion to name a few. Many people experience emptiness; some feel shame and guilt. Some feel gratitude, or a sense of relief. The feelings of grief can last for a long time after the death.

Although grief is not a simple emotional process, it is not in itself an illness. However, grief can occasion illness (Kissane, 1996; Tomarker et al., 2008), particularly when there are complications to grief. Depression is not uncommon, and anxiety disorders may arise, as often as in 20% of caregivers who are grieving (Schulz, Hebert, & Boerner, 2008). Physical illnesses also may accompany the mourning process (Shear, Monk, Houck, Frank, & Reynolds, 2007).

In this chapter, we will begin with a brief discussion of typical hospice bereavement services. We then offer a synopsis of the common view of grief as an individual, personal experience, in contrast to the family systems approach to mourning. Then we will compare a meaning of loss and death in families with family emotional process (FEP) to those with addiction emotional process (AEP). We will detail some of the likely complexities of mourning among members of families with AEP, consider how such complexities can influence mourning, and address the role of recovery in the mourning process. We will provide suggestions as to how hospice bereavement programs might better serve families with AEP.

HOSPICE BEREAVEMENT PROGRAMS

Bereavement program coordinators and others on the hospice team make assessments of how survivors will mourn so they can provide appropriate services. Most often, these services consist of invitations to support groups and periodic inquiries into how the person is doing. The standard time frame for bereavement follow-up is about a year after the death of the loved one. This structure reflects more the requirements of the Hospice Medicare Benefit than the actual course of mourning, which can easily last 2 years and beyond. During the first year, mourners probably do benefit from bereavement support. Yet the second year, when mourners are more likely to begin a practical reengagement in life, is just as important. Generally speaking, however, most hospice bereavement services do not address that period in a mourner's life. In other words, the systems of hospice bereavement support do not fit the realities of many of the mourners that they are intended to support.

According to the National Hospice and Palliative Care Organization (NHPCO), bereavement professionals represent slightly over 4% of the hospice staffing (NHPCO, 2008), which in our opinion is an inadequate number of professionals to address completely the complexities of mourning that families are likely to face. A recent study identified that the stress experienced by adult children, family members, and those care providers who do not live with the dying patient is often overlooked by hospice, and resurfaces with more difficulties in bereavement (Bushfield & Fitzpatrick, 2008).

Furthermore, bereavement assessments may not take into account how variable mourning can be. Generally speaking, predictions as to how an individual or a family will handle the loss of a loved one are made on several specific bases: (a) previous patterns of mourning, (b) present sources of social and familial support, and (c) the individuals' own assessments of how they will mourn.

The difficulty with these parameters is that they are built on presumptions made in the present about past and future needs. They do not take into account the radical changes the survivor experiences. The world as the survivor knew it before the loved one died, vanishes at the moment of death, and is replaced with another world. This new world of life-after-loss may *look* familiar to the one who is grieving, but it is very different indeed.

Furthermore, many factors—the timing of the loss in the life of the survivor; the relationship with the one who has died; concurrent stresses and/or losses; the personality of the one mourning—explain why every person's experience of grief is different. These complexities may be overlooked or oversimplified by hospice's bereavement programs because, again, most hospices are simply not prepared to address the full range of emotions raised by grief over the extended timeline of mourning—nor are they required to by law.

CONTEMPORARY UNDERSTANDINGS OF THE PERSONAL EXPERIENCE OF GRIEF

Contemporary understandings of the phenomenon of human mourning begin with Freud's *Mourning and Melancholia* (1917). However, most modern conceptions of grief were influenced by Kübler-Ross's groundbreaking study, *On Death and Dying* (1969). Although Kübler-Ross later repudiated her use of the term "stages" (Kübler-Ross, 1984), and in spite of the fact that she was not addressing the processes of grief in her book about the experience of terminal illness and dying, "stages" and "grief" became linked in the popular mind. This is regrettable. As two contemporary grief researchers have said: "One result of Dr. Kübler-Ross's work is that many people now tend to apply the concept of stages to other aspects of human emotion. Grief, which follows death, divorce, and other losses, should not, however, be regarded in terms of stages" (James & Friedman, 1998, p. 11).

Applying the concept of "stages" to mourning has at least two unfortunate and misleading results. One is that it leads to a sense that the emotions of mourning follow (or should follow) a particular order, and that the process of mourning should result in an "acceptance" of the loss. We now understand that grief does not actually have "stages," and that whatever "acceptance" of the loss that occurs may not, in itself, bring mourning to an end. The other misleading result of expecting a sequence of emotions is that it takes the focus of mourning away from the transformation of one's relationship with the deceased. As James and Friedman have said, "The nature and intensity of feelings caused by a loss relate to the individuality and uniqueness of the *relationship*" (James & Friedman, 1998, pp. 11–12). Mourning, as with all things having to do with the end of life, is primarily about relationships.

Present-day epistemology in grief, loss, and mourning rests on foundations first articulated by John Bowlby (Fast, 2003). Bowlby, following Freud, postulates that grief is an emotion to experience and "work through" rather than an emotion to circumvent or to pathologize. The implication is that healing from the death of a loved one may not be curable by pharmacological or other medical means alone, but rather that healing requires time and support. In Bowlby's model, human relationships and their attachments are complex, and therefore, so is grief. Length and complexity of mourning are not contingent on age, time spent in a relationship, or interdependence. Rather, all those who love, grieve the loss of a loved one—which makes grief a central part of caring, caregiving, and caretaking.

In a similar vein, Therese Rando suggested that all death experiences incite an incalculable range of emotional responses and intensified physiological distress (1986, p. 21). She identified aspects of mourning that proceed from avoidance of the loss, to confrontation with the impact of the loss, and to reestablishment of normal relationships.

William Worden recognized that mourning was not merely an emotional process but a practical one. He said, "mourning creates tasks that need to be done" (Worden, 1992, p. 38). The "work" of grief necessary for adapting to the loss could be accomplished, he thought, through these four tasks: accepting the reality of the loss, processing the pain of grief, adjusting to a world without the deceased, and finding an enduring connection with the deceased in the midst of embarking on a new life (Worden, 1992). This "task model" of mourning is ratified by Rando. She also recognized that "working through" one's feelings might entail certain "tasks of mourning," including the need to recognize the loss, react to the separation, recollect and re-experience the deceased, relinquish old attachments, readjust to a new world without the deceased, and reinvest energy in new relationships (Rando, 1986).

Rando and others (Cacciatore & Bushfield, 2007) have indicated that there is a long trajectory of grief, and that during bereavement, rather than severing our bonds with the deceased, we need to form a new, yet ongoing relationship with the one who has died. Establishing this new relationship is often challenging, and can be a complicated process for a variety of reasons. Worden (2002) identified a number of mediators to the mourning process, including: the relationship with the deceased; the mode of death; historical aspects, including history of other losses; personality variables; social variables; and concurrent stresses.

Complicated mourning or *complicated grief* manifests in such a way that it interferes significantly with daily functioning. Although complications may emerge during both anticipatory grieving and during bereavement, they are unique experiences (Prigerson, Frank, Kasl, & Reynolds 1995; Tomarken et al., 2008). Complicated grief often includes elements of stress response (Shear et al., 2007), but may also be demonstrated as the complete absence of emotional response (Brintzenhofe-Szoc, Smith, & Zabora, 1999). It is appropriate for persons experiencing complicated mourning to seek psychotherapy as well as support.

We also want to recognize that sometimes, the term *complicated grief* is used in hospice bereavement programs in a way that describes less the grief experience of the mourner, and more the inability of the bereavement program to address the grief of the mourner adequately. In other words, "complicated grief" can be used as a term that means "a grief more complicated than our program can address." Such persons are often referred to psychotherapists and other professionals. But the point is, when "complicated grief" is used in that way, it is less of a *diagnostic* term and more of a term used to describe the limitations of the hospice bereavement program.

McGoldrick, Anderson, and Walsh (1989) identified five questions clinicians consider particularly important to ask those who are dealing with the emotional aftermath of death:

1. What are the culturally prescribed rituals for managing the dying process, the deceased's body, the disposal of the body, and commemoration of the death?
2. What are the family's beliefs about what happens after death?

3. What does the family consider an appropriate emotional expression and integration of the loss?
4. What do they consider to be the gender rules for handling the death?
5. Do certain types of death carry a stigma (e.g., suicide), or are certain types of death especially traumatic for that cultural group (e.g., homicide)?

Each of these authors and researchers shares an appreciation for the significance of *relationships* in mourning. For us, this means that although grief may be an *individual's* emotional experience after loss, no one's grief occurs in a vacuum. Although approaches to personal mourning have made allowances for variations in personality and history, still we remain embedded in contexts larger than ourselves—in cultures, in societies, and in families. It is within these larger relational entities that we grieve, and from these larger relational entities that we learn how to mourn—how to receive support, comfort, and care—so as to be not alone in our loss.

Toward this end, we believe that hospice bereavement programs can better address the emotional needs of survivors if they adopt a *systems* approach to mourning. When a member of a family dies, the whole family, as a system, goes into mourning. When the family member is being served by hospice, this mourning pattern can be anticipated even before the family member dies, as discussed in chapter 6. This systems approach would provide a new perspective on the mourning experience by retaining and maintaining the mourner's context within the family system of which he or she is a member.

DEVELOPING A FAMILY SYSTEMS APPROACH TO MOURNING

As with the process of dying, mourning from a family systems perspective is less a matter of an individual's experience than it is a matter of a system adjusting to an event in its history. To use the language of William Bridges (2004), if the death is the event of *change* for the family, then mourning is the *transition* it makes toward a new homeostasis.

In other words, a death in any family occasions a series of "repositionings" of the members of the family. Because mourning can take an indefinite period of time, this repositioning to achieve a restoration of homeostasis can also go on indefinitely.

One way to imagine what this process might look like is to picture a "stabile," a sculpture of movable parts that remains relatively motionless when not disturbed. In the stabile of the family, death removes one of those parts. The result is a kind of collapse—until the pieces of the stabile are repositioned and a new stability is reached. This repositioning is what occurs as a family mourns.

The ability of a family to achieve a new stability depends on the self-differentiation of its members. In a family whose members are relatively well differentiated, there is less anxiety to bind, and fewer fears of separation or distance. Family members are freer to make their own way through mourning. They are more likely to receive understanding and support from others in the family, less likely to feel judged, and less anxious that their particular methods of grieving might be hurtful or frightening to other family members. A greater degree of mutual respect supports each family member's coming to his or her own terms with the meaning and the impact of the loss. The family can more easily discover a new homeostasis.

Even in the healthiest of families, the levels of self-differentiation are likely to vary, of course. More important for our purposes is the significance of Bowen's multigenerational emotional process to a family's mourning (see Kerr & Bowen, p. 221f). Bowen's sense was that the relative stability or instability in the family system could be "passed down." In his words, "very unstable functioning in one family member is usually associated with unstable functioning in other family members in the existing and preceding few generations. Similarly, very stable functioning in one family member is usually associated with stable functioning in other family members in the existing and preceding few generations" (Kerr & Bowen, 1988, pp. 222–223).

We posit that grief is in itself a de-stabilizing influence on a family's homeostasis. In families that are less well differentiated, as families in AEP tend to be, individuals and the family as a whole simply might not have the "tools" to grieve appropriately and completely. This would mean that with each loss, the family would experience the continual destabilization of its functioning.

In sum, mourning is likely to be more complicated and incomplete for those who are less well-differentiated than for those who are better differentiated. This is why self-differentiation is itself a predictor of

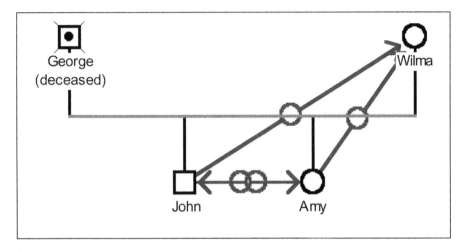

Figure 7.1 The effects of George's death on the Cinnamon family.

whether the complexities of mourning will result in complications—or not. For this reason, a systems approach to bereavement assessment is likely to result in a more appropriate tailoring of bereavement services to family members because it aims at assessing the self-differentiation levels in the family, appreciating both the individuals involved, and how they function together as a family.

Because a death in the family is a de-stabilizing event, it challenges and even threatens the levels of self-differentiation achieved before the death occurred. The transition period of mourning challenges not only the system, but also the individual members of it to maintain their levels of self-differentiation. Some will maintain; others might even improve; and still others may experience a loss in self-differentiation. Through the rise and fall of levels of self-differentiation, the family can make adjustments in its homeostatic balance.

The time it takes for families to make the adjustments in its homeostasis is likely to be beyond even the most discerning hospice bereavement service provider. Figure 7.1 illustrates the pull toward homeostasis after the death of a family member. The bereavement providers would do well to note that Wilma's efforts at rebalancing occur in concert with Amy's and John's. Figure 7.1 helps illustrate the push toward stabilization of the triangle; however, it is by no means a simple act to rebalance or "replace" George in the family triangle.

MOURNING IN FAMILIES
WITH ADDICTION EMOTIONAL PROCESS

For many reasons, families in AEP will likely experience mourning differently than others—from their relationships with other family members to their personal and family histories. One aspect we have mentioned previously is the multiplicity of losses those in AEP are likely to have experienced (Durazzo, Rothlind, Gazdzinski, & Meyerhoff, 2008; Liberto & Oslin, 1997; McGoldrick, Anderson, & Walsh, 1989). Given the length of mourning, let alone its other factors, multiple losses often result in overlapping grief and tend to mean that bereavement will be unresolved. Histories of multiple losses necessarily result in an experience of mourning that is both complicated and incomplete

More important to our discussion are findings that clearly link the lack of differentiation with more complicated grief reactions, especially with respect to anxiety (BrintzenhofeSzoc et al., 1999). Adaptability in families highly influences mourning. Reassigning roles and power, and making shifts in response to particular situations, require a repertoire of adaptive behaviors (McGoldrick, Anderson, & Walsh, 1989; Olson, Portner, & Lavee, 1991). As we have discussed in chapters 5 and 6, families with AEP are likely to exhibit a narrow repertoire of adaptation.

Thus, mourning is more likely to be complicated for those who are less well-differentiated than for those who are better differentiated. In sum, a systems approach to bereavement assessment is likely to result in a more appropriate tailoring of bereavement services to family members. Because it aims at assessing the self-differentiation levels in the family, appreciating both the individuals involved, and how they function together, a systems approach to bereavement can "paint the big picture" of a family's overlapping losses without making the individual members of that family personally responsible for resolving or completing their mourning.

In FEP, the death of a family member is an occasion for a release of anxiety, and that anxiety must now be bound—again—only this time, without the *active* participation of the deceased. The anxiety of grief in FEP can be bound in other ways. For instance, it can be bound to the *memory* of the family member. We witness this often when families continue to take into account the family member who has died. This is *healthy* mourning. Thus families who place flowers on the graves of deceased members, or who remember their birthdays, and even those who speak of them in the present tense or consult with them around family decisions (saying, for example, "What would Mom have wanted?" or "What would Dad have done?")—all are, in their own ways, trying to bind anxiety.

In AEP, shame as well as anxiety must be bound. Just as "shame and death are close-linked," so is shame an aspect of the suffering and pain of the grief that follows death (Schneider, 1977, p. 75). AEP makes us aware that shame is an aspect of all mourning. We find in the mourning of those in AEP, occasions for shame-based thinking, shame-centered feeling, and shame-management behavior, as described in chapter 5.

Families with AEP experience certain *barriers* to effective, complete, and satisfactory mourning. These barriers are related to the "rules" of family life, the multiplicity of previous losses, the multigenerational emotional process, and other, specific experiences related to the phenomenon of addiction.

Rules in Addiction Emotional Process

In chapter 3, we discussed how families with histories of addiction tend to live by three rules: Don't Tell, Don't Feel, and Don't Trust. We have seen how these rules function in AEP (chapter 5) and how they come into play as aspects of caregiving and caretaking (chapter 6). Now we will see how these rules affect how members of families with AEP are able to mourn.

The purpose of these rules is to bind the chronic shame felt by families. With the addition of the acute shame of mourning, the rules are tested. If the rules of family life in AEP function like emotional circuitry, the sheer quantity of emotions in mourning could "overload" them, with the result that their ability to bind the (combined) shame of mourning might be inadequate. Understanding that this can be true for those in *systems* of AEP—that it is a matter of how the system as a whole manages the shame it is experiencing—can help hospice bereavement professionals better understand why, for instance, some members of a family participate in support programs, and others do not. From a systems perspective, it is less a matter of whether one individual "benefits" from that participation, than how that individual's participation benefits the family as a whole. From a systems perspective, the whole family benefits if one member mourns well—and conversely, the truncated or complicated mourning of one can have a deleterious effect on the mourning of others in the family.

Don't Tell

Families in AEP can have strict rules (spoken and unspoken) about what can be talked about—and what cannot. The number of secrets that are kept, who talks to whom and who does not, the level of disclosure, the insulated family life (not letting outsiders know what occurs within the family): All contribute to a higher level of chronic shame, anxiety and fear that the reality of life in the family might become known. In mourning, the impact of the Rule *"Don't Tell"* is not only upon how the family communicates, but also upon *what* they communicate about. Family members may not be aware of what others are thinking, or feeling, or doing, simply because they are not being told.

"Not telling" contributes to the *isolation* members of families in AEP experience with their mourning. The resultant feeling, often, is anger. Resentments build because thoughts and feelings and actions cannot be revealed without breaking the rule. Acting out and acting in occur in lieu of verbalization. Often, anger is easier to release than the shame that underlies it.

In this way, the rule of *"Don't Tell"* can give rise to more tumultuous mourning in a family, as anger substitutes for other feelings. Families in AEP are more likely to exhibit shame as an aspect of their grief: They are likely to be ashamed to be mourning at all; they feel set apart and exposed; they may feel self-conscious, as if "everyone" knows—or should know—that they are in mourning. However, they are likely to be reluctant or even afraid to talk to anyone about their shame or other feelings, since that could entail disclosing aspects of their family life that are likely to be regarded as shameful. Finally, members of families in AEP are more likely to bind their shame in ways that use blame to produce guilt. Thus, in mourning, members of families in AEP are more likely to feel guilty about what was or was not done in the course of providing care for their loved one, or more generally in the course of their lives.

One can easily see from this how inhibitions in the communicative processes of a family can become a barrier to effective grieving. Instead of speaking about what is meaningful to them as individuals, family members are more likely to be aware of topics that must be avoided and to be reticent about speaking about the deceased or the family with the hospice bereavement team. Lacking practice, and sometimes skills, in communication, family members are constricted in their abilities to make decisions and to process the meaning of what they are enduring. Family members may be less likely to turn to each other for support, or to take the view that they are in this mourning together.

Wilma wished there was someone she could talk to about her relationship with George. She wanted to know whether she was wrong to wonder whether George had loved her. She needed reassurance that she had cared well for him, because he never told her that she had. She worried that someone from the hospice had known about her drinking at night, and that maybe that had led to her missing something and George dying "too soon." Looking back over their life together, she worried about what she could have done differently.

But she found it difficult to share her thoughts with anyone. She tried one of the bereavement support groups that Heart of Gold Hospice offered, but all of the other widows there seemed to have had perfect marriages, so she didn't feel she could tell them about what hers was really like. And when she tried to talk with Amy about the family or her care of her father, or anything, really, Amy just got peevish and impatient. Wilma thought about talking with John, but, well, he lived so far away, and when he did come over, she didn't want to ruin his visit by telling him how she was really doing.

Don't Feel

As we have discussed in earlier chapters, expressions of feelings in families with AEP are discouraged. This does not mean that the individuals in the system do not experience feelings. Rather, because shame is bound through the Rule of *"Don't Feel,"* expressing their feelings, even acknowledging their feelings, brings about not only the feeling itself (sadness for example) but also a *shame* response. Breaking the rule of *"Don't Feel"* leads to an unbinding of the shame, and can lead someone to feel ashamed of whatever emotion they feel. A family member may ask: *Is there something wrong with me that I feel this way?* One result of the combination of "*not* talking" and "*not* feeling" is that individuals lose the ability to express feelings appropriately. Consequently, they may distrust their own feelings, and may even rule some out, perhaps telling themselves that they are not supposed to feel the way that they do. This is how there comes to be a kind of *estrangement* within and among family members that is exacerbated during periods of grief. The inhibited nature of the expression of feelings could be its own barrier to effective mourning.

John was astonished with how much emotion he experienced after his father died—about his relationship with his father, about his relationships with his mother and sister, about his family life, about himself as a father and his relationships with his children. He decided to take a special, 3-month seminar on the 12 Steps. The first 3 weeks went by all right, but when he got to the Fourth Step, he realized: There was no way he was going to be able to complete his inventory in a week! Memories came back of things he had long forgotten. The realization dawned over and over again about how much things in his life were interconnected, and influenced each other. John decided to quit the seminar and simply keep working the Fourth Step for as long as it seemed to be needed. He knew he'd get the release and relief of the Fifth Step soon enough.

But it struck him: He felt much closer to his sponsor and his friends in the program than he did to his own family. That's all right, his sponsor told him, there would be time to address that when he did the Eighth and Ninth Steps. When John expressed his surprise that the death of his father would bring out so much of what he was feeling, his sponsor replied, "I guess you didn't realize before that the Steps were about grieving, huh?"

Don't Trust

Perhaps the most damaging rule for living among families in AEP is the rule of "*Don't Trust.*" These families develop a sense of "inside/outside," which can mean that the family becomes its own insulated entity, and "outsiders" are not to be trusted. This adds to their sense of isolation and estrangement. But family members also do not trust each other. Members are never quite sure about what will happen at any given time. A chronic suspiciousness develops.

For members of these families, trusting is risky not just in itself but also because it will likely bring about the release of shame. They are not comfortable with the vulnerability that comes with trusting and they fear the shame that would come from having their trust betrayed.

If one has learned not to talk, feel, or trust, one will have great difficulty processing the many feelings that accompany grief. To whom *would* one talk? Talk about *what* feelings? And could the other be *trusted* with the information? The occasion of a death in the family presents formidable emotional challenges for those who are members of families with AEP.

After her father died, Amy hoped her life would return to normal. She redoubled her efforts to care for her family, fearing that she had neglected them in favor of her father. She wasn't quite sure how she felt when they told her they'd been OK. She wanted to feel missed—more than missed, really. But her kids even said that they had liked their father's cooking! Or at least that they'd had pizza as often as they had....

Amy felt uneasy. She wasn't sure she hadn't "forfeited" her place in her family. She looked at her husband less with gratitude for what he had done while her father was dying, than with suspicion. She wondered how he could still love her if he had found out that he could get along without her. She even found herself worrying that he would leave her.

Amy thought about talking about her feelings with her pastor, but then she decided not to. She knew what had happened to others who had confided in him: Pretty soon everyone in the church knew what was troubling them. She told herself she might as well get up in front of the whole congregation on a Sunday morning and spill her guts! She was resentful and afraid, and thought she better keep it to herself. "This too shall pass," she told herself. But then, it didn't.

Barriers of Previous Losses

Families with AEP are likely to have experienced a greater number of losses than families without histories of addiction, prior to the death in the family. In fact, it has been said that addiction is a "disease of losses," and "living with alcoholism can feel like [one is in] a constant state of mourning" (Al-Anon, 2002, p. 23).

Some of the losses that these families experience are the deaths of other family members, as addiction results in shorter life spans and poorer health. In addition, there are other, less tangible yet no less significant, losses that these families may experience. Some of these are: loss of security, loss of childhood, loss of dreams or of a confidence about the future, and loss of relatedness.

Loss of Security

Whenever AEP is present in a family, there is likely to be a higher level of chaos as well. That chaos could be internal, in terms of the family members' behavior toward one another, or external (for example, in terms of loss of jobs or frequency of moves). The higher level of chaos results a loss of a sense of security. Members of families with AEP learn that their space can be invaded or violated at any time. As a result they often become extremely self-protective or self-oriented, as if they are on their own. It can appear as if "everyone for oneself" is the motto in such families.

Loss of Childhood

Children in substance-abusing families often lose the "role" of child long before chronological adulthood, because they cannot depend on their parents for their physical or emotional needs. A child in a substance-abuse family may feel so compelled to provide for her own sense of safety and security that she views adults' efforts to provide these as infringements on her autonomy (Wheeler, 2003). Children in substance-abuse families come to realize that their parents will not be providing this for them. Of course, mixed signals of role confusion and expectations can occur in any family. However, this is more common for children in families with AEP. For instance, children of addicts often feel the emotional absence and decreased functioning of the parents. They often seek to compensate by assuming parental roles and behaviors. They are highly likely to feel *personally responsible* for their parents' behavior, and may blame themselves for it. The gains in "self-organization" made by children in substance-abusing families come at the price of loss of childhood (Wheeler, 2003).

When a death occurs in a family with AEP, the feeling about the loss of childhood often surfaces and presents itself for mourning.

Loss of Dreams or Future

Sometimes the impact of having lived in an addictive family is so subtle that a family member may not even realize the extent to which they have lost their dreams or visions for the future; they simply stopped dreaming long ago. If the loss of childhood has to do with insecurity about the past, then the loss of the ability to dream has to do with an insecurity about the future. Family members may have difficulty envisioning a life for themselves that is separate from the one who has died.

As we saw above in a vignette about John, mourning this loss of "the dream" is an important aspect of AEP. In most people, the realization of this loss begins early in life, when the child of a family in AEP first experiences the realization that his/her family is "different" from other families. What they had thought was "normal," and thus typical or shared, turns out to be "different." Out of this loss of sense of being "normal" or living in a "normal" family comes the dream that, one day, "being normal" might happen for them.

The irony experienced by those in AEP who are mourning is this: Most who experience mourning hope that, through their grief, some sense of being "normal" might be recovered; normality, life as they knew it to be, might return. For those in AEP, there has already been an experience of the loss of the "normal"—yet, the wish or hope that "normal" might some day be, remains. In their mourning, there is no "normal" to return to, which makes the hope for "normal" through mourning all the more poignant.

Loss of Relatedness

In AEP, a loss of relatedness can occur on several levels. The addict loses his relatedness with the other family members (in favor of the drug of choice) and the family, in turn, loses their relatedness to the addict. But then, this loss cascades among the other members of the family, as each one seeks to discover how to relate not only to the one(s) who is/are using, but also to each other. They lose relatedness to the degree that they focus upon the addict. Just as recovery for the addict is essentially the restoration of a capacity to relate to his own self and other people, so recovery for members of the addict's family means a restoration of an ability to relate to *their* own selves, and to each other—apart from relating to the addict.

This loss of relatedness is shared by all of the members of the family. And, it is likely to become most evident at the time of a death in the family because mourning is a shared emotional process in every family. Families with AEP may find that their interactions are impaired. Their abilities to support and understand each other are limited. More likely, each has been so wounded by the other in the course of their common experience as family that members are likely to retreat into their own emotional processes, in separation and even isolation from other family members.

Addressing the Multiple Losses and Grief of Families in Addiction Emotional Process

The individual family members may be both so acquainted with loss, and so overwhelmed by the multiplicity of the losses experienced, that they may not see the present loss as extraordinary or different. Or, conversely, they may see the present loss as an occasion for mourning all of the other losses the family has experienced. The experience of multiple losses may bring a persistent sense of unresolved grief.

Every loss can be an occasion for the reopening of previous losses. What has not been resolved in the past may become available for resolution in the present—and the resolution that has been achieved can be reexamined and perhaps reworked. In families with AEP, however, the multiplicity of opportunities to mourn does not necessarily bring about an increased sense of confidence in the ability to mourn. New losses produce the opposite of confidence: A *dread* of yet one more loss; or a numbing and a denial of the feelings of grief; or the false hope that all previous mourning might be resolved in just this one. In any case, the hospice bereavement professional can expect a surplus of feelings to result from the presenting loss—whether those feelings are expressed or not.

Hospice bereavement professionals can use a "Loss History" to help themselves appreciate the impact of multiple losses upon the survivors they are supporting. Given the levels of chronic shame present, taking a Loss History requires sensitivity to the significance of the information that is being revealed. But, done well, the Loss History can help family members visualize the multiplicity of their losses—from which they may be encouraged to draw their own conclusions.

A comprehensive Loss History would begin with placing on a time-line the most concrete information about loss and change in the family. Questions such as, "When did your grandparents or parents die?" can lead to others, about where people have lived and worked. Most of the losses named above will not have specific times of occurrence, but the sensitive bereavement professional could list them as questions or include then as categories on a Loss History, for example: *Have you ever had the feeling that you lost your childhood? When did you first have that feeling?*

Guided by dimensions of loss, grief, and bereavement that may provide encouragement and inspiration, as well as information for assessment, a loss inventory which includes aspects which are restorative, evaluative, interpretive, affirmative, affective, and transformative may provide the most complete loss inventory (Dennis, 2008). Examples include the following:

- What previous losses are you aware of?
- How did you make sense of those losses?
- What feelings were you aware of when you experienced each of those losses?
- Were there differences? How might you describe how these differences were experienced?
- Which aspects of the loss you experienced were most troubling? Least troubling?
- After some time had passed, did you notice any changes in how you thought or felt about the loss?
- Were there any positive things that came out of the loss?

A loss history is an exploration; as such, it has both a process and a product. Helping individuals examine and reflect how past losses are re-examined in the face of a new anticipated loss can be helpful in understanding the complexity of grief and loss.

The most important thing for hospice bereavement professionals to remember is that members of families with AEP may experience a shame response as they become aware of the impact their losses have had on their lives. If hospice bereavement professionals recognize this, they can respond appropriately and compassionately, addressing the shame the bereaved are likely expressing. (See chapter 10, where this is addressed more extensively.)

Barriers of Multigenerational Process

In chapter 5, we stated that a family systems approach to addiction fit well with contemporary disease models. We referred to Bowen's work that addresses how systems' emotional processes are likely to replicate or return from one generation to the next.

Nowhere is this phenomenon more significant than in mourning. For the multigenerational nature of both addiction and family emotional process means that the death of a family member in one generation is likely to have an impact upon other family members in other generations—and not merely the one that immediately precedes or follows the death of a family member. A death in any family will bring about a destabilization in its homeostasis. The destabilization following a death in a family with AEP brings with it a release of at least some of the chronic shame that had been previously bound. In addition, the destabilized family must also find some way to manage the acute shame of mourning. This means that, until that chronic shame can be bound again, the family is likely to experience a period of volatility in its emotional process. Most of the time, this volatility is going to be expressed in behaviors, not merely in higher degrees of emotionality. And given the family's history, these behaviors are likely to be addictive in nature.

Barriers Related to the Phenomenon of Addiction

There are certain aspects of the phenomenon of addiction that in themselves present possible barriers to effective mourning. These aspects are physical, as well as psychosocial and/or spiritual.

Depending upon the drug of choice, the physical abilities of the addict to stand and withstand the feelings associated with mourning may be impaired. Further, as mentioned earlier, addicts live in families, which are intolerant of the expression of feelings in general. The physiological result can indeed be an impairment of the nervous system to such a degree that the addict's ability to feel is literally blunted (Kessler et al., 1996). This deadening can complicate mourning.

Psychosocially, families with AEP often experience what can be called an "abandonment in place": People might appear to be present for one another, but their *emotional* availability is likely decreased (Mirin, Weiss, & Griffin, 2002). Further, as mentioned earlier, family members learn early to depend on themselves for everything and to be suspicious of outsiders. Thus these family members are less likely to seek bereavement support, either from professional individuals or from groups. For both of these reasons, family members may be unable to access support from each other or from outsiders.

Family members who have experienced recovery, and have used services such as Alcoholics Anonymous, Narcotics Anonymous, or other support groups, may have unlearned the "don't tell, feel and trust" rules that inhibit bereavement group participation, and may be better able to benefit from support groups. The length and meaningfulness of recovery may mend and alter the psychosocial impact of living in a family with AEP. In this sense, the *spiritual* growth that comes through recovery optimizes the mourning of those individuals.

OVERCOMING BARRIERS TO MOURNING USING A FAMILY SYSTEMS APPROACH

The paradox of taking a family systems approach to mourning is that while the hospice bereavement professional may be in contact with only one member of the family, that person is always to be viewed in the *context* of the family. Still, benefits are to be gained by meeting with as many family members as possible. Let us go back to our example to illustrate.

Jane, the Bereavement Counselor for Heart of Gold Hospice, called Wilma and arranged for a home visit with her, Amy, and Kate (John's ex-wife). Meeting with the three women, Jane asked about Wilma's typical day. She not only listened to Wilma, but she also observed her affect, particularly when Wilma described the late afternoon, a time she spent with George. Describing this time of day, Wilma wept openly.

Amy and Kate seemed surprised by Wilma's weeping. Jane asked whether Amy called Wilma once in awhile, now that George had died? Amy said that she had, but that she hadn't noticed Wilma's sadness. An off-hand remark Kate made about her ex-husband, John, and his drinking, suggested to Jane that perhaps the history of alcohol misuse or even abuse involved more than one generation.

Jane made three suggestions: First, that Amy, John, and Kate create a schedule of daily calls to Wilma, particularly in the late afternoon when Wilma missed George the most. Second, that the three of them (John, Kate, and Amy) pay attention to how well Wilma was eating and taking care of herself. And finally, that Wilma and Amy and Kate, and perhaps John, seek out Al-Anon meetings in their areas, and begin to attend regularly, to deal with the issues of grief, George's addiction, and the addiction in John's family.

This last suggestion surprised Wilma and Amy. Jane noted that neither of them were especially enamored of the prospect of going to Al-Anon. Kate was the only one to say something positive. She volunteered that she had been going to Al-Anon meetings for the past 3 years, and that it had helped her in her relationship with John. "I just hadn't thought about it helping me with my grief, too," she said. Then she thought for a minute, and added, "I'm going to see if Johnny and Serena want to come with me, too."

When Jane returned to the office, she arranged for additional bereavement volunteers for Kate and Amy, and a male volunteer for John.

Let's look at Jane's intervention from a family systems perspective. First of all, Jane did not treat Wilma as an individual apart from her relationships with her children. She did not inquire about the ebb and flow of Wilma's feelings, but about how she spent her time, and she noted which parts of the day were lonelier than others. She included Kate and Amy in the *listening*. To her credit, Amy heard her mother differently than she had before. And Kate disclosed information about John that gave Jane a fuller appreciation of the system. This was a credit to Jane, whose approach did not heighten the shame or otherwise make Amy, Kate or Wilma feel that their family was "different" from other families.

Second, we want to note how gentle Jane was in suggesting possible rearrangements in the family interaction. She made her suggestions in a matter-of-fact way, while addressing the most difficult time in Wilma's day. Jane accepted the history of the family process without feeling tempted to address the emotions themselves. Were the family to be seeking therapy, addressing their emotions and their meanings would be necessary. But for the sake of a bereavement plan of care, a strategic, not a therapeutic, intervention is better. And done gently, as Jane did it, the intervention may be better accepted by the family members—and if accepted and enacted by them, it has a better chance of success.

Finally, Jane did not ignore the role and history of alcoholism in the family. She did not shrink from addressing it directly in her suggestions. Although she was direct, she also presented the positive possibility of Al-Anon as an affirmation or a recognition of what was, not as a consequence to diagnosis of a pathology, or otherwise as an assessment the family might take to be blaming, perhaps triggering a guilt reaction. Done well, the suggestion of 12-Step meetings for dealing with mourning and coming to a better understanding of themselves can open constructive alternatives to members of families with AEP, alternatives they might otherwise even have been afraid of or reluctant to accept for themselves. The evidence of the success of Jane's matter-of-fact presentation can be found in Kate's disclosure of her participation in Al-Anon, dating back to a time preceding John's entry into recovery and further supported by her understanding of the desirability of including her and John's children in the Program.

We would want also to notice what was not said or addressed: The behavior of Johnny and Serena. Kate did not say how they were mourning the death of their grandfather, but because of the multigenerational process, Jane could have assumed that they might be somewhat at risk. Kate's willingness to include them in her Al-Anon meetings now could be a ratification of that assumption. But whatever is occurring in Johnny and Serena's emotional process was not stated. Just because this was not directly disclosed to Jane does not mean that her intervention was inadequate or incomplete. There will always be aspects of a family's life together that bereavement professionals do not know or will not find out about. However, a comprehensive approach to the family as a system will inevitably influence everything about the family's life together—whether the bereavement professional knows about the particular circumstances or not.

In other words, Jane facilitated the family in focusing on the living (Wilma), rearranging their homeostasis (by moving the two siblings together in the hope of mutually supporting their mother), and in providing an opportunity for the family members to learn about and accept their family and its emotional process by meeting others with like histories (through Al-Anon). Moreover, the *community* each family member could find in Al-Anon would be helpful to them beyond their period of mourning for George. Jane's intervention introduced the possibility that their mutual mourning could indeed become a positively transformative time in their family's history. Jane's inclusion of Kate, who, even as the ex-daughter-in-law, was still an integral part of the larger family system, suggests an avenue to transform the family system for the next generation as well.

SUMMARY: MOURNING AS AN OPPORTUNITY FOR TRANSFORMATIONAL CHANGE AND GROWTH

We have discussed some of the challenges faced by members of families with AEP as they enter their periods of mourning following the death of a family member.

Now we want to say a positive word about mourning as an *opportunity* for such families. The period of mourning in any family is an opportunity for the self-differentiation of its members and a challenge to their customary homeostasis. During mourning, most families feel the gravity of the moment as a pull toward belonging. As the family reconfigures itself, and a new homeostasis gradually achieved, the instinctual tensions Bowen describes are both heightened, and tend to favor emotional processes that tend toward belonging and away from individuality. It is for this reason, paradoxically, that self-differentiation—actually, becoming better self-differentiated—becomes all the more possible. That the pull toward togetherness becomes more obvious and observable serves to permit choices for self-differentiation that may not have been previously recognized.

In families with AEP, it is perhaps appropriate to describe the *crisis* of mourning in those terms of the Chinese character, that is, as a time of both "danger" and "opportunity." The process of grief and mourning can mirror that of *recovery*, since recovery describes the detachment and distance not only from the substance of abuse but also from the behaviors that accompany an addictive attachment. In other words, in addiction terms, recovery is one way to gauge self-differentiation.

Recovery is an important concept for several reasons. At a first level, it signifies the level of awareness in the family and its members of the presence of addiction. That a person enters into recovery is itself a gauge of the family member's self-awareness and willingness and ability to pursue self-differentiation.

At a second level, the number of persons in the family who are active in their recovery will be its own gauge of the family's capacity for self-differentiation. This in itself is a fair predictor of how the family will grieve—not how *well* but *how*: that is to say, the *pattern* that they will follow. In mourning, gains toward self-differentiation will be lost or compromised in favor of a return to earlier paths of belonging—including a resumption of addictive behavior, or, in the case of nonaddicts, the codependent enabling from which such persons were in recovery.

If this seems as if we are describing the same process in different terms, it is because we are. Loss, and the challenge of mourning, can be a trigger or precipitating event for those in recovery from addiction. And the challenges to *care*, appropriately, for others—without the loss of self associated with caretaking and codependency—are especially poignant and forceful during mourning. Whereas at other periods in family life, the conflicts associated with becoming our own selves might seem to be abstract, during mourning the duality at the core of FEP is both real and felt.

The opposing possibility is equally evident. If gains of recovery are in danger of being lost, then it is also possible for further gains to be made. For the same palpable manifestation of the tension within FEP accords those in recovery *choices*—and making choices is a self-differentiating capacity, even if the choice made *appears* to support togetherness over self-care. This is because, before recovery, there was a sense of "no choice." One's behavior was ruled by compulsions, and overwhelmed with a sense of helplessness. To know that one has choices; to feel that one is making choices; to take into consideration oneself and the quality of one's relationships with others in the process of making decisions: These are all qualities of recovery that can be enhanced during mourning.

Mourning thus becomes a mirror we can hold up to ourselves, and see in it our possibilities for becoming better persons.

REFERENCES

Al-Anon. (2002). *Opening our hearts, transforming our losses.* New York: Alcoholics Anonymous World Services.

Bridges, W. (2004). *Transitions: Making sense of life's changes* (2nd ed.) Cambridge, MA: Da Capo Press.

BrintzenhofeSzoc, K., Smith, E., & Zabora, J. (1999). Screening to predict complicated grief in spouses of cancer patients. *Cancer Practice, 7*(5), 233–239.

Bushfield, S., & Fitzpatrick, T. (2008, November). *Impact of social work intervention on hospice caregiver strain*. Paper presented at the Gerontological Association of America, Washington, DC.

Cacciatore, J., & Bushfield, S. (2007). Stillbirth: The mother's experience and implications for improving care. *Journal of Social Work in End of Life and Palliative Care, 3*(3), 59–79.

Dennis, M. (2008). The grief account: Dimensions of a contemporary bereavement genre. *Death Studies, 32,* 801–836.

Durazzo, T., Rothlind, J., Gazdzinski, S., & Meyerhoff, D. (2008). The relationship of socio-demographic factors, medical, psychiatric and substance-misuse co-morbidities to neurocognition in short term abstinent alcohol-dependent individuals. *Alcohol, 42*(6), 439–449.

Fast, J. (2003). After Columbine: How people mourn sudden death. *Social Work, 8*(4), 484–488.

Freud, S. (1917). *Mourning and melancholia*. New York: W. W. Norton.

James, J. W., & Friedman, R. (1998). *The grief recovery handbook* (p. 109f). New York: HarperCollins.

Kerr, M., & Bowen, M. (1988). *Family evaluation: An approach based on Bowen theory*. New York: W. W. Norton.

Kessler, R., Nelson, C., McGonagle, K., Edlund, M., Frank, R., & Leaf, R. (1996). The epidemiology of co-occurring addictive and mental disorders: Implications for prevention and service utilization. *American Journal of Orthopsychiatry, 66,* 17–31.

Kissane, D. (1996). Family grief. *British Journal of Psychiatry, 164,* 728–740.

Kosminsky, P. (2007). *Getting back to life when grief won't heal*. New York: McGraw-Hill.

Kübler-Ross, E. (1969). *On death and dying*. New York: Scribner.

Kübler-Ross, E. (1986). *Death: The final stages of growth*. New York: Touchstone.

Liberto, J., & Oslin, D. (1997). Older adults' misuse of alcohol, medicines, and other drugs. *Research and Practice Issues, 13,* 94–112.

McGoldrick, M., Anderson, C., & Walsh, F. (1989). *Women in families: A framework for family therapy*. New York: W. W. Norton.

Miller, N. S., Giannini, A. J., & Gold, M. S. (1992). Suicide risk associated with drug and alcohol addiction. *Cleveland Clinic Journal of Medicine, 59*(5), 535–538.

Mirin, R. M, Weiss, R. D., & Griffin, M. V. (2002). Relationship of treatment outcomes to parental pathology. *British Journal of Addictions, 81,* 777–789.

Olson, D. H., Portner, J., & Lavee, Y. (1991). Family adaptation to stress. *Journal of Marriage and Family Therapy, 53,* 786–798.

Rando, T. (1986). *Loss and anticipatory grief* (p. 24). Lexington, MA: Lexington Books.

Rando, T. (1993). *Treatment of complicated mourning*. Champaign, IL: Research Press.

Schneider, C. D. (1977). *Shame, exposure and privacy*. New York: W. W. Norton.

Schulz, R., Hebert, R. T., & Boerner, K. (2008). Bereavement after caregiving. *Geriatrics, 63*(1), 20–22.

Shear, K., Monk, T., Houck, P., Melhem, N., Frank, E., & Reynolds, C. (2007). An attachment-based model of complicated grief including the role of avoidance. *European Archives of Psychiatry and Clinical Neuroscience, 257*(8), 453–461.

Tomarken, A., Holland, J., Schachter, S., Vanderwerker, L., Zuckerman, E., & Prigerson, H. (2008). Factors of complicated grief pre-death in caregivers of cancer patients. *Psycho-Oncology, 17,* 105–111.

Wheeler, G. (2003). Shame, guilt, and codependency: Dana's world. In R. G. Lee & G. Wheeler (Eds.), *The voice of shame* (p. 203f). Cambridge, MA: Gestalt Press.

Worden, W. (2002). *Grief counseling and grief therapy: A handbook for the mental health practitioner* (3rd ed.). New York: Springer Publishing Company.

8 The Hospice Team as a Family System: Systems Aspects to End-of-Life Care

The Heart of Gold hospice team meets weekly to discuss the patients on their census. The meeting is led by their medical director, Hiram, MD. The staff includes two RNs, in addition to Susan; two social workers, Bill and Josie (who works part time); Jane, the Bereavement Services Coordinator; and Rev. Gene, a retired Protestant minister who provides spiritual care part time. The Hospice Manager, Kathy, attends periodically.

To this point we have made a case for applying family systems theories with families who are receiving end-of-life care. We have pointed out some ways in which a systems approach helps to account for certain emotional dynamics that occur within families, and the impact of family emotional process (FEP) and addiction emotional process (AEP) on the family's response to end-of-life care and bereavement. In this chapter, we will focus on the emotional processes or patterns that may be present in hospice teams. We will discuss how hospice teams function in many ways that are similar to families; we will examine the emotional processes of the hospice team; we will discuss how grief and mourning in particular can have an impact upon the functioning of the hospice team; and finally, we will discuss effective leadership of hospice teams.

THE HOSPICE TEAM AS "FAMILY"

Hospice professionals commonly speak of their team as a "family." This sense of family acknowledges both the coordinated effort it takes to provide care, and the sense that the individual hospice professionals are participating in a *system* that transcends their individual expertise and efforts, with its accompanying emotional processes.

Both of these observations were affirmed by Edwin Friedman, a family therapist and ordained rabbi, when he wrote:

> Family theory can be applied to all work systems, depending primarily on two factors: (1) the degree of emotional interdependence in that relationship system and (2) the extent to which its business is 'life'....[W]ork systems that deal with the basic stresses of life, particularly medical...partnerships,...are particularly susceptible to the rules of family process, including those rules that govern who in the family is likely to become ill. (Friedman, 1985, p. 197)

We believe that hospice teams meet both of these criteria, and they do so in ways that are distinctly different from other health care provider relationships. For instance, hospice teams tend to be "closed" systems, since there is a need for continuity on the team, to ensure consistent care. For that reason hospice teams strive for limited shifts in personnel, and promote a sense of sharing in the endeavor of care. This heightened sense of belonging and the resulting need to balance or harmonize one's individual skills and personality to and for the good of the whole, tend to make the hospice team a "family"-like system.

In this way, hospice teams typically display the high degree of "emotional interdependence" that Friedman names as his first criteria for applying family systems theories (Friedman, 1985). There is mutual positive regard, and consideration is given not just to the differing levels of skill among persons on the team, but also to the variable levels of emotional availability. For instance, one team member may have a more difficult time participating in the service of a particular patient or family; thus the team will adjust however it can. Or, perhaps one team member has been especially affected by the series of deaths experienced among the patients or families under his/her care. Attuned to the impact of grief and accrued losses, the team will attempt to adjust. These adjustments are likely made "on the fly," in the course of their life together as a team, and often without self-critical review. That is, the team seldom stops to question how one team member's emotional functioning has an impact upon the others. Teams adapt, but most often simply accept, unexamined, the consequences of the emotional interdependence of the team-as-system. This parallels family life, wherein more often than not similar dynamics and emotional processes go unexamined.

Friedman's second criterion also applies to the hospice team as "family," in that the business of hospice is the business of life and death. There is an ongoing awareness among members of the hospice team that they are participating in the life-shaping transitions of their patients and families. This awareness lends an emotional richness to their work. Many hospice professionals sense that their work affects them personally—by providing end-of-life care, their own lives are affected. Serving on a hospice team is not merely a job for which one receives a performance evaluation. For the hospice professional providing end-of-life care, the very humanity of the personal/vocational interface demands a deeper appreciation of emotional processes. Hospice staff recognize the meaning that this gives to their own lives (Ablett, 2007; Hospice Management Advisor, 2007).

Beyond Friedman's criteria, there are other ways in which hospice teams can be described in family-systems terms. For instance, hospice teams are interdisciplinary. This means that a mutual respect of disciplines, perspectives, terminology, and personalities different from one's own needs to occur in order for the team to function well. Because of this, it could be said that the team's ethos promotes self-differentiation, even as consensus over care must be reached. Hospice teams mimic families in the tension between individualism and belonging; but they also differ from most families in that they typically lean toward and encourage self-differentiation.

The team needs its members to bring different perspectives and professional skills to bear. In terms of ideal team functioning, this means that the team depends on each of its members living up to her/his *role* on the team. This in turn has two consequences. On the one hand, team members are compelled to relate to one another. Although emotional cutoffs, for example, are possible in families, they are not possible on hospice teams, and to the extent that they do occur, the results are far from beneficial. This to say that professional roles prescribe a starting point for hospice team members, but these professional identities alone do not help hospice professionals know how to relate—they must develop patterns of relatedness within their specific teams.

On the other hand, hospice professionals often experience unclear boundaries. Nurses may find themselves asked by patients or families to provide spiritual care; spiritual caregivers are asked for help with family and psychosocial issues; and social workers are often asked to explain medical information or to perform nursing services. The permeable nature of the boundaries among the professions on the hospice team parallels how families function, and lends a sense that every team has an identity and life of its own, just as every family does.

These are just some of the general aspects of the emotional processes of the hospice team that parallel those in our personal families. In the next section we will explore four specific aspects of team functioning in family systems terms: homeostasis; triangles; overfunctioning; and self-differentiation.

APPLYING A FAMILY SYSTEMS
APPROACH TO THE HOSPICE TEAM

When we construe the hospice team as a "family," many of the family systems concepts introduced in chapter 4 can be applied to the team's functioning. In work teams, as in our personal families, family systems' terms are descriptors of how *anxiety* is being handled. Another word for "anxiety" in work teams is "stress." The recognition of "workplace stress" is common to all types of businesses. Hospice teams members must function with levels of stress—perhaps chronic stress—in attending to the needs of their patients and families as well as the needs of their team members. If we can translate the psychological term of "anxiety" that Bowen uses to describe FEP (Kerr & Bowen, 1988) into the term "stress" to describe how anxiety is experienced and processed in a hospice team, then, we might better understand the "family-like" emotional processes of the team.

Stress originates from many sources, and individuals handle stress in different ways. But because our perspective regards the system as a whole, we are interested in how the *system* adjusts to stress. We are interested especially in the ways the system adjusts to individual ways of adapting to stress—just as we were interested in how the family system adjusts to the individual ways its members bind their anxiety.

That is, just as families have their own emotional process, there is what we refer to as *team emotional process* (TEP). Just as FEP entails how family members think, feel, and behave, TEP entails how team members think, feel, and behave. Moreover, just as "belonging" to one family or another influences one's own emotional process, belonging to one hospice team or another influences one's own TEP.

FEP is similar to TEP in the following way. To manage the stress within the team, members have at least three choices to maintain homeostasis: they may form triangles, or they may overfunction, or they may become more self-differentiated. Consequently, here we will discuss these key concepts and how they function within TEP.

Homeostasis

Susan, RN, had the longest tenure with Heart of Gold of any of the nursing staff. She had watched as Heart of Gold's average daily census grew from the mid-20s into the 40s. Now, as it stretched toward 50, she knew that increased caseloads were to be expected. So, when George's case came to the team for admission, she was not surprised when Dr. Hiram (affectionately called "Dr. Hi" by the team) turned to her and said, "Susan, I'm assigning this patient to you. Is that OK?" Before she could answer, Dr. Hi turned to Bill, and said, with his head down, "And of course, Bill, since you work with Susan with many of her patients, you will want to see what you can do with George Cinnamon, too." Bill nodded.

Even though she had tacitly accepted adding George to her caseload, Susan made a mental note. She had told herself before the meeting began that she already had a full caseload, one that was larger than the other RNs'; she had promised herself she would refuse more patients. But she didn't act on her promise. And she kept to herself her feelings about working longer hours than the other RNs, along with the fact that the two of them had caseloads significantly lower than hers.

Hospice teams, like families, seek balance and resist alterations to the balance they have achieved. However, in hospice, as in all businesses and families, change is a constant. Homeostasis is the principle that lets a system's limitations in adaptability to change be recognized without attributing those limitations to the resistance or reluctance of individual persons within the system. Typical challenges to a hospice homeostasis might be changes in personnel, or changes in caseloads and average daily census. Homeostasis is nearly always maintained at a cost—and the price for that maintenance is often not apparent to those charged with keeping the hospice team's balance. Hospice professionals have noted that the shifting emphasis in hospice from its spiritual purpose of *caring* to its business mission of *profitability* is a challenge to the team—in particular, to its homeostasis (*U.S. News and World Report*, July 21, 2008).

In the above vignette, we can see one aspect of how Heart of Gold is maintaining its homeostasis in a time of change. As the organization attempts to increase its census and thus grow its profitability, its TEP is affected. George Cinnamon is just one of several new patients coming onto service. These patients must be assigned to someone—at least to a nurse and a social worker. As the medical director, Dr. Hi makes these assignments proficiently. And on the surface, they are accepted, in accordance perhaps with a professional resignation to the realities of the situation. Thus the homeostasis of the team's emotional process is maintained and unruffled.

But we are also getting a first glimpse at how Susan is "binding" the stress of the TEP—and the challenge that this is to her own emotional process. We will illustrate this interaction further in the following sections.

Triangles

After Susan and Bill, MSW, admitted George, they walked to their cars together. Along the way, they found themselves discussing how things were going on the Team. Susan admitted that she was working longer hours, and that sometimes those hours wore on her. Bill was somewhat surprised to hear it. Like the others on the Team, he had come to regard Susan as a "super nurse." Respecting her confidentiality, Bill said nothing to anyone about the stress Susan felt she was under, nor about what he saw to be her growing resentments toward the other nursing staff.

As in FEP, homeostasis in TEP is maintained, lost, and regained through triangles—the interlocking relationships that exist in all sys-

tems. In families both natural and vocational, triangles are the structures of homeostasis. Through them flow the emotional processes that
determine how content issues are managed. As within families, triangles
in TEP can exist among people, issues, and/or behavior. Triangles can
include external factors, such as caseloads, and internal factors, such
as self-image. Moreover, in chapter 9 we will see that triangles can
include persons and issues *not* readily apparent to the team, such as
family matters or family members of team members, or even matters
or relationships from team members' pasts.

   In FEP, triangles are evidence of how anxiety is being bound. That
is, triangles serve to stabilize the anxiety among family members. In
a similar way, within TEP, triangles represent a functional structure
that serves to maintain homeostasis and manage stress. When alliances
are forged among three members of the team (just as in a family), or
with an object, in the case of George and Wilma's "triangle" with happy
hour, these identifiable triangles may function to provide a reliable
structure to manage stress. In chapter 4, we discussed how triangles
operate to manage anxiety in families. In teams, they function similarly
with regard to stress.

   In an effort to bind the anxiety or manage the stress of TEP,
triangles become the often unrecognized or unidentified structures of
homeostasis. For instance, it is easy to see in the Heart of Gold Hospice
the alliances among the threee team members: Dr. Hiram, Susan, RN,
and Bill, the Social Worker, in how they function in team meetings.
The easy and assumptive level of communication among these three
testifies not only to their professionalism, but also to the special bond
that has arisen in the course of their years of working together. They
are familiar with one another.

   This presents difficulties to the team, however. On the one hand,
their assurance in their interactions can exclude other members of the
team from voicing their ideas and opinions. And on the other hand,
such traditional patterns can inhibit even those who are participating
in them from voicing their own internal concerns. TEP achieves its
stability at the price of this lack of self-disclosure.

   To understand how triangles get formed in TEP—and in FEP, for
that matter—we would do well to distinguish between "triangles" as
a noun that describes structures in systems and "triangulation" as a
behavior or activity through which triangles are formed.

For example, we have noted that Dr. Hi, Susan, and Bill have formed a triangle in the course of their having worked together over the years. There may or may not have been any *intentional* activity of triangulation that brought that triangle to be. Yet out of that triangle, another has been formed, this one among Susan and Bill, and Susan's *image* on the team as a "super nurse." Again, whether it was intentional or not, the very nature of the conversation between Susan and Bill "triangulated" the two of them with Susan's need to uphold her image as "super nurse." This created a new structure in the TEP. In all probability, the team's emotional process was already exhibiting this triangle, since the team relied on Susan's sense of herself as a "super nurse" in order to function as it did in managing the stress of increasing the census. Still, that triangle was tacit, or implicit in the team's functioning. Susan's request for confidentiality or her otherwise relying on Bill not to tell anyone what she had told him, reveals the way the triangle was already functioning in the team's emotional process. Through such actions as Susan bringing Bill into her confidence, both implicit as well as explicit triangles may develop. In chapter 9 we will see how confidences among team members can have the same impact on TEP as "secret-keeping" does in AEP.

To understand the impact of the activity of triangulation in the shaping of structural triangles in TEP, we can speak in terms of "triangling *in*" and "triangling *out*." For instance, on the one hand Bill found himself "triangled *in*" around Susan and the Hospice Team's image of her as the "super nurse." Bill was reluctant to address what it would mean for the Team's functioning if Susan were to step out of that role.

On the other hand, Susan "triangled" Bill *out*—because her confiding in him led to her having a particular trust in him, which singled him out from other team members. She felt Bill could keep her confidence as a "secret" about how she felt about work and how she felt about the other nurses. This led to an alliance that separated Bill out from the Team. Susan looked at Bill as a likely ally, should she ever choose to address the situation with the Team or with administration.

In other words, the triangles of TEP serve to shape that process. They are indicative of the ways that stress is being managed among the team members. As alliances, triangles speak to emotional attachments and lead to boundaries that are generally more rigid, as we can see with how Susan and Bill more frequently work with each other with certain hospice patients, like George Cinnamon. But these triangles can also indicate how team members have become separated from others on the team. The "special relationship" among Susan and Bill and Dr. Hi serves to exclude others and to separate Bill from the other RNs with whom he must work as part of the larger interdisciplinary team.

From this observation, we can see that what begins as a triangle in one situation results in other triangles forming—much like repeating family patterns. To illustrate this and other relationships within the team, we use a figuring device patterned on the genogram that we have called the *teamogram*. A teamogram differs from an organizational chart. The teamogram maps not an official hierarchy, but rather the connections and parallel emotional processes that exist among and between the team members and the family they serve.

Figure 8.1 shows these triangles within the team relationships. In Figure 8.1, we can see both the structural triangle of Dr. Hi, Susan, and Bill (indicated by the bold line connecting them), and the "triangulation" of Bill and Susan with the "super nurse" image (indicated by the shaded triangle that is filling the space among and between them).

Overfunctioning

The confidence that Susan and Bill shared contributed to their choosing to work more frequently with each other. As more patients came on service, Bill would volunteer to work with Susan. (Dr. Hi, noticing this, reinforced the pattern with his assignments.) Bill found he preferred seeing the patients he and Susan were working with together over some of the other RNs' patients and families.

This in turn had other consequences. Josie, the other social worker on the team, began to be preferred by the other nurses, in part because they could count on Josie seeing their patients without having to be prompted. Josie did not question her growing caseload: She saw herself as someone who was more capable and could simply get more work done efficiently.

Within a system's understanding of FEP, when members of the family system attempt to maintain homeostasis, it requires each member of the system to fulfill his or her part. When one member does not fulfill his or her part, another member must step in and overfunction to keep the system operating. Likewise, if one member overfunctions,

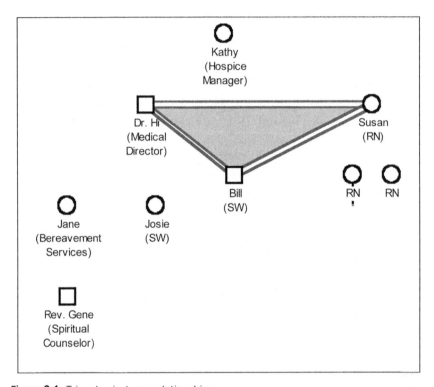

Figure 8.1 Triangles in team relationships.

other members of the system can underfunction. In this way, "uneven" or "unbalanced" systems still balance themselves.

Similar balance-through-unbalanced participation operates in the functioning of TEP. Susan and Josie show signs of overfunctioning; their working harder allows the hospice team to maintain its homeostasis. They give good *reasons* for overfunctioning, and each receives some reward for his or her behavior: Susan, from the hospice management and from patients who request her; Josie, from the other nurses. Their overfunctioning reinforces the way they either like to be seen (Susan) or like to see themselves (Josie). Neither is particularly aware of how her overfunctioning affects the overall emotional process of the hospice team and contributes to the maintenance of its homeostasis—which at this point is actually an *im*balance among the nurses and the social workers.

Hospice teams have been studied very little. Research has indicated, however, that hospice staff identify certain "work climate" issues, such as social support, participating in decisions, and reasonable workloads, as associated with reduced stress among staff (Vachon, 1999). These factors suggest a balanced distribution of both work and support for that work—features that are elements of a team's emotional process. However, teams may "balance" themselves overall through having some members overfunction in order to compensate for the underfunctioning of others. When Susan works harder (takes on more cases) than others on the team, it may be in response to others "not pulling their weight," but the result is that by taking on more work, Susan temporarily stabilizes whatever tension might arise around this imbalance—no one need address who is "not pulling his/her weight" or otherwise notice the imbalance of the workload among nurses on the team. A "well balanced team," therefore, might well consist of over- and under-functioning members, in equal parts.

How and why such balancing-by-imbalance arises in TEP can be explained not just in terms of accepted work practices. More likely, these are patterns of behavior learned in childhood, just as coping styles developed in childhood tend to inform adult coping strategies (Hawkins, Howard, & Oyebode, 2006). In other words, this is one way that our personal family's emotional process influences the emotional process of any team of which we are a member.

One insidious aspect of overfunctioning in hospice teams is that it often brings praise or positive reinforcement from the overfunctioner's employer and colleagues, just as Susan generally received positive reinforcement from Dr. Hi and Kathy, the hospice manager. What remains unexamined is the question of whether or not it is *healthy*, either for the employee or for the system as a whole. Friedman (1985) suggests that the same rules that govern family process, such as who in the family is likely to be ill or scapegoated, may apply to the team's functioning. Within the Heart of Gold hospice team, the unspoken expectation is that Susan will continue to work as she does and that she will not become symptomatic or ill. Should an overfunctioner's health deteriorate, the emotional process of the team will be affected. The homeostasis of the TEP will need to be restored in some other way.

Unfortunately, it usually takes a health crisis on the part of an overfunctioner for the team to alter its emotional process. This might seem unfair, or at least preventable: It might seem logical simply to delegate patient care equitably. However, this is easier said than done—precisely because the team's functioning is an *emotional* process. For instance, what would it mean to the Heart of Gold hospice team's emotional process if one of the other RNs insisted on staying within his/her manageable caseload limits, even when Susan was exceeding hers at times of need? One could say that this nurse was exercising her abilities at self-definition—but others on the team might see her as less of a "team player" and might be less inclined to reward her with positive regard for her behavior. That nurse could be seen as "not pulling her weight." As it was, for Susan, the positive regard as "super nurse" was so important to her that she in effect depended on the underfunctioning of the team's other RNs in order to preserve the status and respect she obtained from her overfunctioning.

Overfunctioning may contribute to the homeostatic balance of a team's emotional process, but it may also lead to other problems on the team, just as it does in families. We will discuss these problems more completely in chapter 9.

In hospice teams the stresses of providing end-of-life care are nearly always bound to have affects on those providing it. Yet there is, just as frequently, a lack of recognition among those participating in the system of how the functioning of the system itself is "shaping" them—in terms of their physical, mental, and emotional health and behaviors.

Self-Differentiation

Hospice professionals have identified certain struggles in their work together (Parry, 2001). Many of these struggles relate to the roles and boundaries on the interdisciplinary team, as well as the stress of competing demands in hospice care. Similar to the life course of families, team members bring histories to their collective interaction and to their attempts to manage the stress that arises in their work. Just as in families, togetherness and separateness compete *within* us, to challenge our levels of self-differentiation, as well as *between* us, to produce anxiety when our belonging is threatened. Team members experience the competing forces of both wanting to belong and to feel a part of the "team" and wanting also to maintain their own personal and professional integrity in their work together.

Hospice nurses in particular identify struggles with the balance between closeness and distance, and describe boundary-setting as one means to maintain distance that allows them to function effectively in their professional role (Blomberg, 2007). Within the team, professional roles can assist with distancing and self-differentiation, by more clearly defining *who* is to do *what*. The success of this role differentiation, however, is variable. At their best, interdisciplinary teams provide a certain synergy and the various disciplines are enhanced by the knowledge and skills of the others. At their worst, interdisciplinary teams may struggle with "turf battles" when roles are either unclear or overly rigid.

In studying hospice teams, Ablett (2007) noted that certain strengths help mitigate the tensions of hospice work. In particular, one of these personal strengths is an awareness of boundaries and an ability to use boundaries effectively. Since it serves to foster resilience in hospice work, the suggestion is that this strength is an aspect of self-differentiation. Ablett (2007) also discovered that hospice professionals who had a sense of coherence between their own and their hospice's values related to work, death, caregiving, and spirituality were more likely to endure in hospice work.

Contributing to TEP, the individual members of the team each brings her or his own pattern of *personal* emotional process to the management of her or his stress, and to how the team as a whole manages its stress. Often members of hospice teams seek to manage their stress individually. However, the success of their individual efforts actually depends on how they fit within the team's emotional process. This is because work-related stress has a function within the *system* of the hospice team, and therefore, systemic or team adjustments are necessary, not only in order to rebalance team functioning, but also to support team members in their own stress management.

At the time he became George's social worker, Bill was stressed by his increased caseload. The pressure to take on more patients led him to spend less "quality time" with each. So as George progressed through his dying process, Bill felt constrained. He could not simply "be" with George, as he would have liked. And he disliked it when he felt his job was reduced to providing merely functional services for patients and families—like arranging for grab-bar installations or home care worker referrals. Caught between what he found meaningful about his work and the stresses of an increased caseload, Bill capitulated reluctantly to the necessities of time-management.

Heart of Gold Hospice had gone through periods of growth before; in fact, Bill had started his work as a part-time employee. As his caseload grew, gradually his hours were expanded and a full time position was created for him. Similarly, over the years, consistent workload increases eventually led to the hiring of Josie, a second social worker.

What helped Bill alter his way of doing social work were two things. On the one hand, he hoped that the increased caseloads everyone was experiencing as the Hospice's census expanded would indeed be only temporary, as they had been before. Kathy had told him her goal was to be able to hire another SW, even if it were only part-time. On the other hand, he had come to Heart of Gold Hospice because he appreciated their slogan. It read, "Our mission is to provide heart-felt care to everyone: Our patients, their families and our employees." He identified with this because he saw himself as providing heart-felt care.

In FEP, self-differentiation is descriptive of one's ability both to be oneself and yet to belong; to stay emotionally connected with one's family. Each of us achieves our own level of self-differentiation within our families.

However, for many reasons, the level of self-differentiation we achieve in our families is not directly transferable to the other systems in which we, as individuals, participate. First, we *choose* the other systems, as well as how we will participate in them. The roles we have, for example, on our hospice teams—even though they may be limited by our professions—are expressions of these personal choices. How we function in our professional roles may be quite different from how we function in the roles we occupy in our families—or they may be similar.

Second, the systems in which we work may be more or less as well self-differentiated as those of our families. It is likely that our work systems are going to be *better* differentiated—but that likelihood is based on higher degrees of education and certain professional requirements for emotional maturity, which may not hold true in all circumstances.

Third, as in personal family systems, the emotional processes of work systems generally go unexamined or unacknowledged, but the consequences of this lack of examination are somewhat different. That

is, even in work as feeling-oriented, and thought-demanding, and be-
havior-challenging as end-of-life care, the veneer of professionalism
masks, more often than not, the complexity of these elements and
their effects on individual team members. Members of hospice teams
often experience a disparity between the functioning of their personal
FEP and that of their TEP.

For these reasons one can find oneself experiencing a different
level of self-differentiation in one's work system than in one's family
system—and thus having a different experience of one's self! Not
surprisingly, in professional systems such as hospices, people often
have a *better* experience of themselves at work than they do in life.
They can come to feel more competent and more capable, less mired
in the emotional processes of their families. This experience of self-
differentiation is its own seduction: being at work can be more appeal-
ing than being at home (vanDaalen, 2009).

There are two qualities of self-differentiation that hospice team
functioning requires that are especially worthy of mention. First, it
helps to appreciate the complexity of the emotional processes being
manifested if one remembers that end-of-life care is very personal work.
That is, end-of-life caring demands a level of "presence"—emotional
availability—that many other endeavors do not. This is, in part, what
makes the system of the hospice team an existential parallel to the
family system: It matters how they *care*—for others, for each other,
and for themselves.

Yet it is in this rising to this level of caring that members of the
hospice team are especially vulnerable (Morrison, 2009; vanDaalen,
2009). On the one hand, because hospice professionals must be emotionally available, it is almost impossible for them not to bring their
work home; they take their own emotional process wherever they go.
One's professional experiences are carried back into one's home life
and into one's personal family. On the other hand, the reverse is also
likely to be true: One is likely to bring his or her *family* life to work.
One might be able to distinguish between his/her FEP and his/her
TEP—but, ultimately, for each person it is always *one* continuous
emotional process.

The other quality of self-differentiation on the hospice team that
is especially evocative is the capacity to find meaning, even in the
midst of stress and higher degrees of emotionality. Because of the
predominance of the medical model in end-of-life care provision, the

value of meaning and purpose often goes unappreciated, and for that reason is underutilized. The personal care of hospice requires a higher degree of self-differentiation, so that one is better able to attend to one's own needs, the needs of one's own personal family, and the needs of the family being cared for in hospice work—all the while maintaining necessary boundaries between each realm. As Friedman (1985) indicated, the life and death "business" of hospice warrants the need for this self-differentiation so that the TEP may function more effectively. We will address the importance of this capacity for meaning-making in end-of-life professionals in chapter 10.

GRIEF AND MOURNING AMONG A HOSPICE TEAM

If Bill were being challenged to be the sort of social worker he wanted to be with his patients by the higher number of patients he was being required to see, he also was being challenged by circumstances in his personal life. His father was dying, in the care of another hospice service, in another state. Often as he went through a workday, he would find himself speaking with a patient as he wished he could speak with his father. In addition, Bill monitored his father's progress daily, so that he would know better when to take off from work to be with him. He told himself he would use his professional expertise to time it "just right"—and to limit the time he had to spend with his siblings.

Of all of the emotions that hospice teams must process, individually and collectively, perhaps the most persistent, insistent, and telling of the team's emotional process is how it handles grief and mourning. As in families, the manner in which a hospice team mourns very much turns on the degree of self-differentiation of its members.

There are several aspects of the mourning of a hospice team that are different from those in family life. First, and perhaps most obviously, mourning is a constant state for hospice teams, whereas it may seem to be a more infrequent occasion in the lives of families. One could say that mourning is an aspect of or contributes to the chronic stress of the hospice team. To an even greater extent than in many other professions, how a hospice team mourns will determine the quality of its life together. That is, collective mourning is a significant dimension of TEP. One can easily say that a hospice team that mourns together stays together—and experiences a sense of "togetherness" that is both emotionally and vocationally gratifying.

Second, the difficulties many hospice teams face pertain less to their collective mourning—as almost all teams set aside some time for this in team meetings and in the course of the year—and more to their *individual* mourning. As systems, hospice teams depend upon and often assume a degree of self-care on the part of their participants. In general, it is fair to say that hospice teams presume that each member is mourning competently well in her or his own way—without knowing, or trying to find out, really, what that way might be! This presumption leads to another, which is that the level of mourning among the hospice team is relatively constant, or at least bearable, both individually and collectively. Whereas, in truth, the intensities of mourning in each team member, and thus among the hospice team, varies greatly. Mourning as an aspect of all team's homeostatic balance and variables in individual's mourning are yet another aspect of what can go unrecognized and thus unaddressed in the team's emotional process.

Third, as a professional system, and a system of professionals, these presumptions of individual competence and personal attention are often fed by definitions of what it means to *be* "professional." There is at the very least an expectation that one will have learned, in the course of one's end-of-life care experience, how to deal with death, and how to mourn. This may be the case, or, it may not be. For the deaths of individual patients, and the mourning of particular families, may affect us either more than we realize—or more than we are willing to admit.

Moreover, as we have been underscoring, the confluence of emotional processes between one's personal and one's professional lives brings about unique instances of mourning. As is happening in Bill's life, hospice team members experience death within their own families, or suffer other losses or illnesses. Given the nature of end-of-life care, with its desired and perhaps required level of emotional availability on the part of hospice team members for the patients and families hospice serves, it is more than understandable that personal mourning would mix with professional mourning, each having some influence upon the other. As systems, hospice teams are challenged to become adept at balancing these emotional processes as well.

For all of these reasons, the team of Heart of Gold Hospice and other end-of-life care teams benefit from the challenges of providing end-of-life care when their leadership *leads.*

LEADERSHIP TO TRANSFORM TEAM FUNCTIONING

As the Hospice Manager, Kathy purposefully did not attend every team meeting. She meant for her actions to communicate a confidence in the team's ability to manage itself. At the same time, she would occasionally drop-in to meetings arbitrarily. At such times, she would intentionally remind the team that she was available for more than just scheduling issues. She felt she was relatively in touch.

She was surprised then, when she finally learned about Susan's being overburdened by her schedule—and witnessed the lack of response by other members of the team. As the team discussed case after case on the schedule, with Susan as the reporting nurse, Kathy observed that the others had little to say. Moreover, when Josie tried to insert her suggestions, Susan discounted them and turned to Bill for his input.

Noticing this, Kathy mentioned the need to re-adjust some of the case assignments. This prompted Bill to say, without thinking, "It's about time—I was afraid we were burning Susan out!" Kathy noticed the glare coming toward Bill from Susan, who became uncharacteristically quiet. Immediately after the team meeting ended, Susan came to Kathy and told her, in confidence, "I'm really worried about Bill. You know, his father is dying and I'm not sure he is handling it very well."

In chapter 4, we discussed how anxiety arises in family systems because of the tension between wanting to be oneself and wanting to belong. Here we can emphasize that one mark of being a well-differentiated person is to be able to belong in a nonanxious way. If anxiety is a measure of the threat to individuality that belonging entails, then the balance between belonging with others and being oneself can be gauged by the degree to which one participates in a family nonanxiously. This in effect gauges the degree of self-differentiation an individual has achieved within a personal family system.

Similarly, leadership may be defined as being a "nonanxious presence" while providing the necessary authority to preserve the "work" or goals of the team. Of course, it may be easier to think of leadership as a concept that pertains more to work systems than to families. In families, "leadership" may seem to happen by default, courtesy of the hierarchy of the generations. Thus, often within family therapy the goal is to strengthen the leadership function by supporting the authority of the parental subsystem (Aponte, 2001). Too often, parental leadership is confused with parental authority, which in turn can be exercised in an arbitrary way, serving to undermine other functions, such as nurturance or support. More ideally, parents find a way to exercise their leadership and responsibility while at the same time instilling leadership in their children, so that they may come to function autonomously. Ideally, self-differentiation in parents engenders self-differentiation in children. This occurs best when parents can be "nonanxious" about their children becoming independent.

From a manager's perspective, a similar challenge may exist: How do I support the independence of each member of the team, while fulfilling my responsibility to manage the outcomes? Too often, for many managers, as it is for many parents, "leadership" becomes a struggle for control. Yet leaders are more successful, just as parents are, when matters of control are joined in terms of being a nonanxious presence. This is demonstrated by the ability to experience conflict as less of a threat, and more as an opportunity to guide the tension between "all for one and one for all" and "my way is best."

"Leadership as nonanxious presence" can at first glance seem to be an abstract concept, but the "three paradoxes" of Malcolm Payne can help us make it more concrete. Payne (2001) advises:

1. We are to concentrate on building team relationships, but we are not to become so inward-looking and obsessed by the group or our own behavior that we do not look outward, and forget that we are here to serve;
2. Many people value teams as a source of mutual support, yet this support is not passive; it exists for the purpose of building a team, and teamwork is the instrument for carrying out the organization's objectives;
3. Teamwork causes us to focus on our colleagues and our interactions, yet our purpose is not served merely by adjusting to our teammates; instead, our services should be responsive to the service user's needs.

Thus leadership as nonanxious presence means constantly trying to balance these inward and outward foci, as well as the competing forces of constructing a more "managed" team, versus a more "collaborative" team. To do this well, a leader must work constantly on his/her own self-differentiation. Becoming better differentiated means that one is more concerned with one's being a nonanxious presence in the system than with one's authority over the participants in the system.

From a systems perspective, this might be described as the contrast between an open and a closed system. In an open system, the leader is more concerned with the effective functioning of the ever-changing system, than with maintaining an established homeostasis. In either case, effective balance on the team must not become stagnation, or simply a maintaining of the status quo. Leadership as nonanxious presence encourages the incorporation of new team members, new outlooks, and new procedures when needed.

A frequent challenge to hospice team leadership is the triangulation that occurs within TEP. Triangulation often presents itself in personnel matters. Managers can find themselves, for example, embroiled in settling disputes among team members, or in handling requests for assignments. Leadership is needed in managing these professional relationships. Understanding the family systems dynamic of triangles and triangulation can be helpful in assessing and intervening with team members—and in doing so in a way that contributes to everyone's self-differentiation. One knows when this has been achieved when intervention is done in a way that is perceived to be less authoritarian or arbitrary.

Overfunctioning or underfunctioning and other performance issues likewise present critical challenges to team leadership. It is the skilled leader who can recognize how these performance indicators suggest more than "bottom line" financial impact: The overperforming or underperforming team member has an impact beyond the individual's merit performance or customer service outcomes. Just as in families, various team members serve functional roles within their performance parameters. Leadership requires an understanding of how these dynamics are interconnected, and are not solely the responsibility of an individual team member.

The best indicator of a leader's ability to be nonanxious is, of course, how he or she responds to stress. How the leader responds to stress often determines how the team will respond to stress. Certainly, leadership entails a willingness to pay attention, for example, to how various members of the team are "pulled in" to different challenging issues and situations. Being observant, combined with an understanding of how the team communicates and relates to each other, as well as to the families and external customers they serve, guides team leaders in accommodating the various needs of the team in different situations. By the same token, it is the high-functioning team that can look at itself with the same objectivity that it looks at the families being served in hospice care. Leadership as nonanxious presence models this sort of objectivity.

Kathy put a new item on the team agenda for the following week. Her "Director's Report," she indicated, would require a bit more time. Kathy started by acknowledging the good work the team was performing, particularly during the recent growth in census. She described her plan for advertising for two new part-time positions in clinical services, and one part-time "marketing person" to help ensure steady growth and maintenance of their workload.

Then she turned her attention to the team. "We have been working so hard to take care of our patients that perhaps we have not included time in team meetings to address how we ourselves are doing. And we want to be sure that the quality of our care to families is not compromised. I've noticed that we have had some difficult patients, and many deaths; and several of you have postponed your vacations to help us out. I want to be sure that we have temporary staff available to cover our increased workload, so that each of you has the time off you need and deserve. And I'd like to set aside time at each team meeting for us to talk about how we are doing as a team. This may take some practice, but I think it will help us in the long run."

The struggle to maintain balance between economic viability and quality of care is common in hospice (Bradshaw, 1996; Ward & Gordon, 2006). As pressures increase to see more patients in less time, the humanistic core of hospice may be eroded (Ward & Gordon, 2006). Moreover, the temptation to prioritize clinical care over psychosocial care in times of stress can itself produce its own stress. This may be less noticeable to the patients and families that hospice serves than it is to the hospice clinicians providing the service. As Bill's experience illustrates, prioritizing clinical care over psychosocial care can be one source of stress within the hospice team. How that stress influences the TEP warrants attention, and the team's leadership has an important role in addressing this—*within* the team. Reducing stress serves to improve team functioning overall, and to improve the quality of hospice services provided to families at the end of life. But stress reduction is itself more of a psychosocial and spiritual intervention than a clinical one.

SUMMARY

In conclusion, leadership influences not just the system of the team, but its individual members as well. When the leader promotes healthy, self-differentiated TEP, it brings forward the opportunity for reduced anxiety among the team members to be carried back to their families. Just as workers bring their *family emotional process* to the workplace, *team emotional process* may be taken back to the family, where help can well be needed to diffuse and bind anxiety. The boundaries of these two meta-systems have received little attention. But in chapter 9, we will use our understanding of *addiction emotional process* and recovery to understand better how these two larger systems interact.

REFERENCES

Ablett, J. (2007). Resilience and well-being in palliative care staff: A qualitative study of hospice nurses. *Psycho-Oncology, 16*(8), 733–740.

Aponte, H. (2001). *Structural therapy with Dr. Harry Aponte.* Boston: Allyn & Bacon.

Blomberg, K. (2007). Closeness and distance: A way of handling difficult situations in daily care. *Journal of Clinical Nursing, 16*(2), 244–254.

Bradshaw, A. (1996). The spiritual dimension of hospice: The secularization of an ideal. *Social Science and Medicine, 43,* 409–419.

Brandon, E. (2008, July 21). How rising prices impact elder care. *U.S. News and World Report,* pp. 1–2.

Hawkins, A., Howard, R., & Oyebode, J. (2006). Stress and coping in hospice nursing staff: The impact of attachment styles. *Psycho-Oncology, 16*(6), 563–572.

Hospice Management Advisor. (2007). Provide meaning to patients referred at the end of life. *Hospice Management Advisor, 12*(10), 111–113.

Kerr, M., & Bowen, M. (1988). *Family evaluation: An approach based on Bowen theory.* New York: W. W. Norton.

Morrison, R. (2009). Are women tending and befriending in the workplace? Gender differences in the relationship between workplace friendships and organizational outcomes. *Sex Roles, 60*(1/2), 1–13.

Parry, J. (2001). *Social work theory and practice with the terminally ill.* New York: Haworth Press.

Payne, M. (2001). *Modern social work theory.* Chicago: Lyceum.

Vachon, M. L. (1999). Reflections on the history of occupational stress in hospice/ palliative care. *Hospice Journal, 14*, 229–246.

vanDaalen, G. (2009). Emotional exhaustion and mental health problems among employees doing "people work": The impact of job demands, job resources and family-to-work conflict. *International Archives of Occupational & Environmental Health, 82*(3), 291–303.

Ward, E., & Gordon, A. (2006). Looming threats to the intimate bond in hospice care? Economic and organizational pressures in the case study of a hospice. *Omega, 54*(1), 1–18.

9   Hospice Teams and Addiction Emotional Process

Of all of the people on the Heart of Gold Hospice team, Susan is the most candid about her experience with addiction. Because she is not shy, everyone knows her ex-husband was a "hopeless alcoholic."

    Susan is an excellent nurse. She connects easily with families—just walks right in and makes herself at home. Her patients always ask for her, and get quite upset when she sends a substitute. George, in particular, really liked being with Susan. "Just like family," he used to say. George liked to think he knew all about her. She had told him some wild stories about the troubles she had over the years! Susan always seemed to be able to laugh about it—and make George laugh, too.

    In chapter 8, we discussed the connection between the personal and vocational emotional processes of end-of-life care professionals. We described *team emotional process* (TEP) and its management of stress. We discussed the ways that TEP is similar to *family emotional process* (FEP) and its binding of anxiety. Now we are ready to take the implications of this connection a step further.

    In this chapter, we will address how the dynamics of addiction and recovery might influence any team's emotional process, as well as how those dynamics might influence its care of hospice patients and families—especially those with histories of addiction. We will see how the prevalence of addiction among health care professionals may increase the likelihood for *addiction emotional process* (AEP) to exist as an aspect of TEP; how AEP might operate within hospice teams; and how parallel processes function within the hospice team and the families they serve to require shame management as an aspect of end-of-life care. Finally, we will discuss the ways in which the process of being in recovery can have a positive influence on the hospice team's emotional process.

THE PREVALENCE OF ADDICTION EMOTIONAL PROCESS IN HEALTH CARE PROFESSIONALS

Edwin Friedman suggested that, given the "spiral nature of systems" (Friedman, 1985, p. 194), religious institutions tend to function like families. He showed how, in such situations, three levels of the professional's family "plug into one another" in an emotionally interlocking way: one's family of origin, one's present family, and the "family" of the institution (Friedman, 1985, p. 195). We have also followed Friedman's suggestion that since hospice teams exhibit a "degree of emotional interdependency" and are systems whose "business is 'life' " (Friedman, 1985, p. 197), hospice teams experience a similar "emotional interlock."

This means that each person on the hospice team experiences the confluence of emotional processes of their families of origin, their present families, and the "family" of the team. Because their work also asks them to participate in the family systems of their patients, they bring those emotional processes to their life together as a team as well. From this we can easily see that providing end-of-life care is, for the professional caregiver, an exceedingly complex emotional process.

Given the complexity of emotional process of the hospice team, we recognize that addiction emotional process can enter into the team emotional process from essentially four sources: The family of origin of the one providing end-of-life care; the present, personal family system of that person; the prevalence of addiction among persons on the hospice team; and/or through interactions with families with AEP for whom the team is providing care.

Because the presence of AEP among health care professionals influences the emotional process of the hospice team, the principles and perspectives of AEP, discussed in chapter 5, can also be applied within TEP. Throughout, we want to be clear that we are not concerned with identifying addicts or singling out persons (although in our vignettes we will highlight individual's behaviors). Rather, ours is a *systems* perspective that focuses on how the team functions when AEP is present.

HISTORIES OF ADDICTION IN HOSPICE PROFESSIONALS

Addiction emotional process can influence TEP when team members have experienced AEP in their families of origin. Addiction is prevalent in the general population—estimated at 17%, or one of every 15 adults, and recognized as often underidentified and underreported, according to the Substance Abuse and Mental Health Services Administration (SAMHSA, 2007). Addiction is known to be present in the workplace. SAMHSA (2007) estimates 500 million lost days of work productivity resulting from addiction issues. People with family members who have addiction are themselves more likely to have mental health problems such as depression or anxiety (Lambie & Sias, 2005). This supports our premise that addiction in one family member has an impact on the entire family system. Addiction as an aspect of family life leads to AEP as an aspect of that family's life.

It is possible that AEP has an impact on the professions chosen by members of such families. For instance, in the course of speaking about shame, the Whiteheads (1995) made the following observation:

> Children growing up in such a hostile setting [as an abusive family] are likely to...become very adept at 'people pleasing' tactics. We seek out a service career—*ministry, health care, counseling*. Or we marry a partner we can care for full time. Our selfless behavior looks virtuous to us and other people, at least until we recognize its compulsive force. Then comes a stark confrontation with the underlying shame that propels so much of what we do. (Whitehead & Whitehead, 1995, pp. 96–97, emphasis added)

The possibility toward a tendency for AEP to be brought to the hospice team from the families of origin of those serving on the team has been substantiated by research. Among the population of people drawn to the caregiving professions such as those represented on the hospice team, there is a high incidence of family histories of addiction and/or chemical dependency (Baldisseri, 2007).

Nurses had a documented rate of substance abuse of 32% in a study by Trinkoff and Storr (1998), which also indicated higher rates of addiction among certain specialties, such as oncology. Among physicians, there is a likelihood of at least the same rate of addiction as the general population (11–15%), but they are five times more likely to abuse opioids and benzodiazepines—drugs commonly used in end-of-life care—than other substances (Cicala, 2003).

Generally, substance abuse is thought to occur in health care professionals at roughly the same rate of incidence as with the general population; thus, it has been estimated that approximately 10–15% of health care professionals have substance-abuse problems (Dewees, 2006). However, some estimates are much higher—ranging up to 58% (Raistock, Russell, Tober, & Tindale, 2008). The exact prevalence is difficult to determine. Although it could be that the rates of addiction among medical personnel are similar to that of the general population, it is more likely that this rate is grossly underestimated because medical professionals have greater access to controlled substances, and they work in high-stress environments (Baldisseri, 2007; Raistock, Russell, Tober, & Tinsdale, 2008). Some estimate that the rates of use of certain drugs, such as alcohol, opiates, and benzodiazepines, may be 5 times higher among health care professionals (Cicala, 2003).

As with anyone, a hospice professional's chemical dependency can occur at any age. For many health care professionals, however, substance use, misuse, and abuse tends to begin in the course of professional education (Raistock et al., 2008). Addiction is thought to flourish in situations that combine high performance expectations with a low degree of structure (Carnes, 2001)—in other words, precisely in conditions like the work environment of hospice.

Health care professionals may be even more reluctant than others to seek treatment for fear of consequences (Fletcher & Ronis, 2005), and may be very good at hiding signs and symptoms of substance abuse. Programs for the treatment of impaired health care professionals have been established; the most successful ones combine follow-up monitoring and testing along with traditional therapies (Merlo & Gold, 2008). Recovery rates vary but are higher among professionals than the general public; the mixed reviews on relapse rates range from 20–38% or more (Fletcher, 2001; Jones, 2008).

There are many factors that may jeopardize a health care professional's recovery and contribute to relapse. These include: Failure to understand and accept the illness, continued denial, a dysfunctional family, poor mechanisms to cope with stress, overconfidence, poor relationship skills, shame and guilt, and lack of follow-up care and monitoring (Baldisseri, 2007; Fletcher & Ronis, 2005; Gallegos, Veit, Wilson, Porter, & Talbott, 1988; Talbott & Martin, 1991). The number of additional factors that may lead to relapse—such as complacency, self-pity, inability to accept feedback, isolation, manipulation, setting unrealistic goals, and not attending support meetings (Baldisseri, 2007; Tallbott & Martin, 1991)—suggests that a variety of both internal and external factors are required to support recovery from addiction.

Programs for impaired professionals are designed to ensure that they may be rehabilitated and return to work (Baldisseri, 2007). Most health care professionals who re-enter work following treatment return to specialty areas of less stress. Curiously, hospice is often thought to be one of these "less stressful" work environments (White & McClellan, 2008). Yet hospice has several features that may make it undesirable for those truly seeking support and rehabilitation: Accessibility to opioids, a less structured environment; and the compounding of stress due to chronic exposure to grief, loss, death, and mourning, to name a few. Thus hospice service may actually present opportunities for negative consequence to successful addiction treatment and recovery.

ADDICTION EMOTIONAL PROCESS IN END-OF-LIFE CARE

There are aspects of end-of-life care itself that have parallels with the experience of AEP. For instance, hospice professionals' regular exposure to death and its accompanying grief, loss, and mourning can be daunting in terms of the emotional challenges presented. Whether or not individual members of the hospice team grieve these multiple losses, in turn, influences the emotional process of the entire team. The multiplicity of loss faced by hospice professionals is similar to that experienced by families with AEP.

The culture of end-of-life care, dealing as it does with death and dying, is a medical culture set apart from the mainstream. Unlike other health care professions, hospice professionals work in an environment where care, not cure, is the goal. This shift in focus has consequences to TEP.

First, unlike most other medical professionals, hospice team members are faced with the challenges of prevailing cultural attitudes toward death—and the common, accompanying cultural stigmatization. If the experience of death and dying is an occasion for acute shame, then it can be said that the hospice professional works in an environment in which shame could be considered a *chronic* condition. One aspect of AEP on the hospice team has to do with how this chronic shame is managed.

Second, the managing of shame also entails how hospice work is regarded by others. Common misperceptions about hospice care are reflected in the thinking that hospice is involved in "euthanasia," "killing" their patients, or otherwise ending their lives prematurely. Other misperceptions of hospice include the belief that hospice is only for people who have "given up" on living or on whom medical care has "given up." At the same time, there is often expressed a kind of admiration for those providing hospice care. People say to hospice professionals: "How can you *do* that work? I could never *do* it!" The work itself may be stigmatized.

Next we will see how the presence of addiction, AEP, and recovery might be manifested or displayed on the hospice team.

ADDICTION EMOTIONAL PROCESS AMONG THE HOSPICE TEAM

Speaking about the presence of addiction within the hospice team is difficult because it entails addressing personal experiences and emotional dynamics that are stigmatized in our society. Shame inhibits the discussion, yet it is precisely this aspect of the emotional process that requires identification and management. In that sense, shame management is likely to be as important to team functioning as stress management. On the other hand, managing shame in ways that are not shaming themselves is a little practiced art because the presence of shame is underidentified. Accordingly, hospice teams' shame-management skills tend to be underdeveloped.

In this section we will articulate some of the signs and symptoms of AEP as an aspect of TEP, and illustrate how shame can be manifested and expressed. Our aim is to "take the shame out of shame" by appreciating shame and its occurrence in TEP. Our premise is always that from a systems point of view, what one expresses, we all experience. The vignettes about the individuals on the Heart of Gold hospice team are meant to illustrate how the team as a whole is influenced by one person's participation.

Susan had lived with addiction her whole life. Her earliest memory was of cleaning up her mother who had vomited all over the living room rug and passed out on the sofa. She remembered how carefully she washed and scrubbed and tried to make her mother look presentable before her father arrived home.

Later, in her marriage, she was always fixing what her husband had "messed up" while he was drinking. Until she went to Al-Anon, she was determined not to let anyone know what she was really dealing with.

It bears remembering that, in our family lives, AEP is a means for managing anxiety and establishing homeostasis, typically through a set of roles, rules, and relationships. This is also true of TEP.

For instance, the roles that health care professionals tended to play in their families of origin often come to have some influence on their professional choices. Remembering that a hospice professional does not have to *be* an addict to participate in AEP, the same structure of roles, rules, and relationships from one's personal life may be carried over into one's professional life.

The phenomenon of these parallel processes is not in itself detrimental to team functioning. People in caregiving professions (nursing, social work, clergy) often describe their "passion" for their work (Burke & Fikrenbaum, 2009). Interestingly, the link between passion and "addiction" has been established within health care professions (Burke & Fikrenbaum, 2009), and similarities noted between the high commitment and focus on work among health care workers and the "object focus" of addiction (described in chapter 5). In systems where AEP is likely, participants might be seeking to replicate the patterns of behavior that have brought a sense of stability in the past—even when, in the case of addiction, these patterns had their own negative consequences.

By the same token, this means that some professionals who participate in TEP—those whose families have low or no histories of addiction—may be unfamiliar with the ways that roles, rules and relationships *work* within AEP. For that matter, even those who do have a history of personal addiction emotional process might also be unaware of the impact of these roles, rules and relationships on the work environment. In fact, the literature often equates "professionalism" with roles, rules, and relational boundaries (Malleck, 2004; Martinez, 2002; Stone, 2008).

AEP might have enabled the personal family of the hospice professional to function as well as it could. But AEP is disruptive of professional TEP. This is why shame management is a necessary aspect of TEP: Because when a team allows AEP to be exercised unexamined, it forsakes the task of managing shame, and in the process, undermines its own emotional process.

Roles and Addiction Emotional Process on the Hospice Team

AEP in the personal lives of members of the hospice team may have led them to choose prescribed roles, such as "heroes" or "enablers." In a parallel fashion these roles can be manifested in the hospice team, and for the same function—to bind shame. Difficulty occurs when those roles become rigid and persistent because the team functioning reinforces them.

In the example from the Heart of Gold Hospice, we can see Susan bringing to her workplace the patterns of roles that "worked" in her family system. The team may not know this; Susan may not even be aware of this herself. But in her family, Susan became the "super child," the parentified child. By being the "super nurse" of the hospice team, she enacts a familiar role. She also comes to have a stake in being the "super nurse." She fears being "discovered" to be only human. She carries resentments toward her colleague nurses on the team, all the while feeling compelled to function as the "super nurse." These are all symptoms of AEP.

Of course, Susan would not be able to continue to be the team's "super nurse" without the cooperation and tacit consent of the rest of the team. In a way, the hospice team *depends* on Susan to be the team's "super nurse" so that the team can continue to function in an efficient manner. Thus any shame that Susan might be feeling is prevented from being brought forward for discussion and addressed by the hospice team as a whole.

Rules and Addiction Emotional Process on the Hospice Team

Hospice team members who have lived in families with AEP are likely to be aware of the "rules" common to those families: "Don't Feel," "Don't Tell," and "Don't Trust." These rules serve to bind shame in one's personal family system, and they tend to get carried over into TEP to be "practiced" in the workplace for the same reason. Of course, this has consequences for TEP.

Don't Feel

Commonly, within the hospice team, sharing of feelings may be viewed as "unprofessional." Although professional training may indeed have emphasized the need to keep personal feelings to oneself, such instruction is often presented without adequate training on how to accomplish this goal, particularly in the end-of-life care environment where emotions may run high.

The result is that many hospice professionals do not see room within TEP for managing their feelings. They can come to be ashamed of feeling what they do, as they do. The rule of "Don't Tell" instructs them to manage their shame privately. When a hospice team's emotional process includes the explicit or implicit instruction that feelings are not to be expressed, then that team's emotional process is manifesting AEP.

Bill told no one on the hospice team how he felt about his father's impending death. He didn't feel right mentioning it in team meetings because he took it to be a personal matter. Bill got the impression that everyone expected he would just keep on working, but would also do what he needed to do when the time came.

Don't Tell

Where there is "secret-keeping," patient care may suffer and inappropriate boundary violations may occur. Confidentiality is a standard of practice within the hospice team. But AEP brings the difficulty of distinguishing between appropriate confidences and inappropriate secret-keeping.

For instance, recall from the last chapter that Susan shared information about herself with Bill. She asked that he keep it confidential. But that request was, in effect, a request to keep a *secret* because it had less to do with Susan's personal life and more to do with her functioning on the hospice team. We can identify this communication as a "secret," not a "confidence" on three counts: its content included feelings about the other nurses on the team; it triangulated Bill with Susan's team image as a "super nurse;" and Bill felt uncomfortable with having received the information and being asked not to disclose it. Whenever shame is involved, a secret, not a confidence, has been kept, and AEP has come to influence TEP.

Don't Trust

End-of-life care in hospice is an interdisciplinary and interdependent endeavor. The aspect of AEP that most threatens TEP occurs when one team member behaves as if he/she doesn't trust. This can occur in a number of ways: One can develop as sense of "ownership" of patients, to the point that one does not trust colleagues with one's "own" patients. Or one can endeavor to "control" the care provided, to the point that one does not trust family members to provide the care they can. Often when this happens, team members come to see themselves as the "only" one from the team who can adequately care for a particular patient or family. Or one can take such a singular interest in a patient's care that one gets overinvolved. Accompanying this sense of privileged position and its consequent isolation is a tendency to ignore information about the family's emotional process that might otherwise be helpful to the patient's care.

Susan really liked George. She looked forward to her visits with him, and found herself spending disproportionately more time with him than with her other patients. She even scheduled her visits with George at the end of her day, in case she wanted to linger at his home rather than leaving for her own. Whereas many of the nurses talked about their struggles in teaching family members to provide certain aspects of care, Susan simply found it easier just to perform the care herself. Wilma was hesitant at first to turn over so much of George's care to Susan, but soon she began to welcome Susan's visits.

From this we can see how Susan began practicing in isolation from the team's emotional process through her sense of "ownership" of the Cinnamon family, her taking control of George's care, and her overinvolvement with both George and Wilma. Ironically, this isolating behavior stemming from not trusting was one aspect of why Susan became perceived as a "super nurse," because she never reported to the team having any difficulties caring for her patients or teaching end-of-life care to family members. From this example, we can see how, when there is little trust, team fragmentation and professional isolation are likely to occur.

RELATIONSHIPS AND ADDICTION EMOTIONAL PROCESS ON THE HOSPICE TEAM

There are three primary ways in which AEP influences relationships on hospice teams: boundaries, caretaking, and personalization.

Boundary Setting Versus Boundary Violation

The ability to establish relationships is key to end-of-life care. This is, generally speaking, an underappreciated professional skill. For hospice TEP to function optimally, cooperative relationships must be established among and across disciplines and appropriate relationships must be established with patients and family members relatively quickly and easily.

The recognized means for establishing these relationships is boundaries. Boundaries define a professional's functioning, and provide guidelines for relationships among team members, as well as between team members and families. In systems terms, boundaries provide bases for self-definition.

On the one hand, boundaries provide professional identity. On the other hand, in hospice care teams, boundaries may become blurred. They need to be both firm and flexible.

To return to our example, compared to others on the team, Susan easily and readily forms close relationships with her patients. But she does this through personal disclosure: Her patients know as much (or more) about her personal life as she does theirs. Even though this is a boundary violation, for some families, it also works. It can be a familiar pattern of relating that serves a function within that family's system, and may be repeated on the hospice team.

Although hospice TEP would not be well served by rigid boundaries, boundary-testing and boundary-violating are characteristic of AEP. When boundaries are violated frequently, shame results. Thus, for the sake of shame-management, boundary awareness should be pursued.

In the example of Susan's patterns of establishing relationships with the patients and families she serves, the hospice team would serve itself well by asking whether these relationships do not come about as a consequence of the AEP in the families Susan is serving. Perhaps their AEP meshes with Susan's AEP in a way that facilitates relationship establishment, but at the price of inappropriate boundary blurring. Susan's example leads us to wonder whether hospice teams that do not wrestle with issues of boundary setting might be capitulating to AEP within the team's emotional process. When this happens, instead of shame being managed, it simply is ignored.

Caregiving Versus Caretaking in Team Emotional Process

One of the most frequent boundary violations of TEP occurs when caregiving becomes caretaking (as described in chapter 6). The tendency toward caretaking often originates in the original family of the hospice professional. We can easily imagine that this was true for Susan, for example.

Certain characteristics of caretaking in a professional context parallel those in a personal context. Professional caretakers take extraordinary responsibility for the well-being of others, in large part because their own sense of well-being depends on it. They prioritize the needs of others to the detriment of themselves; will feel compelled to provide care, rather than seeing that they have choices in care management; and will engage in denial about the outcome of their provision of care (i.e., death and the end of caretaking). Especially in a professional context, caretaking includes a quality of the *control* one feels. In end-of-life care, the irony is that caretaking is evidenced in the attempts to control the *process* of dying—because, after all, one cannot control the outcome. This is one consequence of the shift in focus from cure to care: the end-of-life professional's caretaking shifts from outcome to process, but retains a similar level of concern with control.

Caretaking on a hospice team may be exhibited in some of the following ways: By a team member's overinvolvement with a particular patient or family; in the inability to "team manage" a patient and/or family; in the expression of having an unreasonable sense of power to control the patient's care; and the way in which a team member may overidentify with one person in the family, to the point of losing objectivity regarding decisions about care.

Evidence that the line between caregiving and caretaking has been crossed signals the presence of AEP as an aspect of TEP. Hospice teams that do not address the caretaking behavior in their emotional process are reinforcing the AEP in their system and de-emphasizing the interdisciplinary cooperation necessary for optimal end-of-life care.

Too often hospice teams allow and even encourage caretaking because it removes a level of decision making from the team's emotional process. For instance, the Heart of Gold hospice team "let" Susan take so many patients as her own. They "gave" Susan a chance to be seen as "super nurse." But Susan's possessiveness caused her stress and worked against her seeking relief from the team's emotional process. It isolated her from the team.

The challenge of AEP to the team's emotional process is to move away from caretaking and toward caregiving. When end-of-life care is influenced by AEP, the team may find itself having to curtail or challenge the caretaking being done by one of its members. The appropriate limits and boundaries of the professional hospice team are designed to be enforced, precisely when AEP would likely ignore or repudiate them.

The intimate caregiving of hospice presents unique challenges for professional care with respect to relationships. End-of-life care has been described as "caring, while letting go" (Thornburg, Schim, Paige, & Grubaugh, 2008). This is as true for hospice professionals as it is for family members. Caretaking entails an unwillingness to let go. The caregiving of optimal hospice TEP encourages sharing in the privilege and the burden of end-of-life care.

Personalization in Team Emotional Process

A tendency toward *personalization* represents yet another parallel between AEP in families and AEP in teams.

In the process of personalization, shame, blame, and guilt function together on the team in a fashion similar to the way they function in families (see chapter 5). For those with AEP, it is difficult to separate being found guilty of a faulty *action* from being discovered to be a faulty *person*. The shame-felt reaction is then a *personalization* of the matter at hand. When a team member's emotional process cannot distinguish between an assessment of an action and an assessment of himself or herself as a person, his or her defensive reaction can be an expression of AEP.

The reaction is likely to be misunderstood. The individual is likely told not to take the matter personally—in other words, personalization brings its own shaming response, in which the individual is shamed for their reactivity, instead of examining the basis for reactivity itself, and addressing it.

Personalization, and the reactivity it displays, is in itself a sign and symptom of the presence of AEP in TEP. Often degrees of personalization prevent aspects of team emotional process, and even procedural concerns, from being addressed in order to avoid anticipated reactivity. The Heart of Gold hospice team, for example, did not think it wise to address Susan's professional conduct with the Cinnamon family. They "knew" she would be highly defensive about it, and they simply did not want to add that experience to any team meeting.

A hospice team's emotional process that is appropriately sensitive to shame-management challenges will see personalization as the evidence that it is in the presence of AEP, and will find ways to address behavior without evoking shame by implying guilt.

MAPPING THE PARALLEL PROCESSES OF END-OF-LIFE CARE

To this point, we have largely spoken about the ways that AEP becomes the concern of TEP. Now we want to speak to how serving a family with AEP can influence TEP.

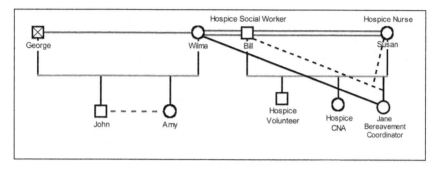

Figure 9.1 Cinnamon family and Heart of Gold hospice team as parallel families.

Sometimes a family's AEP will intersect with AEP already present in the team. Because this was the case with the Cinnamon family and the Heart of Gold hospice team, we can use teamograms to illustrate this connection. But even when the influences and the connections between addiction emotional processes are less clear, they can be noted and used profitably by hospice teams for understanding their own functioning.

We will now discuss four common hospice team issues that reflect an intersection of the team's and the family's AEP. These four common team issues may be evident, in particular, because they run parallel to the patient/family's AEP.

In each instance, we will describe the issue and tell a story about it using an example from the Heart of Gold hospice team. Next, we will illustrate the relationship using the teamogram. As we said in chapter 8, a teamogram differs from an organizational chart. The teamogram maps not an official hierarchy, but rather the connections and parallel emotional processes that exist among and between the team members and the family they serve.

To begin, the Heart of Gold hospice team, in relationship to George and Wilma's family, can be illustrated using the teamogram seen in Figure 9.1. We have placed those hospice workers known to the family on the line between Wilma and George, as "other relationships," and the other, invisible members of the hospice team connected with Susan and Bill and the others, but directly with George and Wilma, in the "parallel family" located to the right. In this way, we can see that the hospice team members' relationship with the family contributes to the family system, similarly to the way additional family members would.

Now we are ready to map the four aspects of AEP that arise from the Cinnamon family and intersect with the AEP on the hospice team: belonging, grief and loss, boundary issues, and shame-sensitivity or awareness.

Belonging to the Emotional Process of the Family

We have said that the ability of hospice team members to establish meaningful relationships quickly with family members is a noteworthy professional skill. By the same token, for some families it is important for them to make hospice team members feel "at home." Sometimes this exceeds hospitality, and families begin to treat hospice team members as members also of their own families. For their part, hospice team members can find themselves identifying with certain members of the family they are serving, which in turn tends to blur one's professional judgment. The hospice team member can decide whether he or she is more a member of the hospice team or the family.

As the team began its meeting, Susan arrived a few minutes late. She explained her tardiness by reporting on George and his family: "I was at the house until after 11 p.m. last night. Wilma and I sat at George's bedside, and I encouraged Wilma to take some deep breaths. George was gurgling, and I could see it was upsetting to her. But Bill and I had gone over all of this with her. She was prepared for his death, but I hated to leave."

Susan wasn't surprised to hear Dr. Hi's report that George had died during the night. But she was concerned that Bill began coughing and left the room briefly.

Developing a sense of belonging to the families they serve results in identification with them and an emotional reactivity, not just to events in their lives, but also to how they are perceived by the hospice team. When a hospice team member responds to a family's overtures to "belong" to that family, that team member is likely to respond in team meetings as if they are in fact members of that family. An emotional intersection has occurred that has consequences for both the family and the hospice team, because it violates the basic boundary of hospice

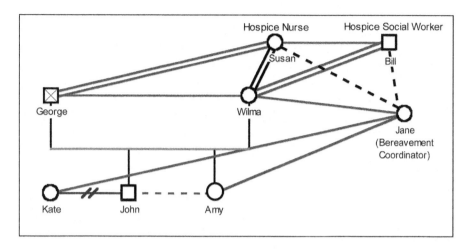

Figure 9.2 Team emotional processes: belonging.

care—the boundary that exists between the team and the family. This violation is itself evidence of an intersection of AEP and TEP.

Figure 9.2 illustrates some of the ways in which Bill and Susan have reacted to the death of George. It illustrates emotional process among Wilma, Amy, Kate, and Jane in order to contrast it with that among Susan, Bill and Wilma. It also illustrates the "connections" between Susan and George, and the "connection" that Bill has established with Wilma. The double lines that link hospice members with individuals in the family demonstrate these connections.

Grief and Loss Issues

The multitude of losses common to families with AEP and to members of hospice teams often results in an intersection of emotional processes that can have an impact on particular members of the hospice team at particular times, as George's death affected Bill.

Bill had tried hard to "manage" the impending death of his father. After all, he told himself, "I know how to deal with this—it shouldn't interfere with my work." But the morning he learned about George's death in the team meeting, he felt tears well up. He began coughing, and excused himself from the meeting.

As he returned to the team meeting, he felt very embarrassed. "Now they are really going to know I've lost it," he thought. However, he was pleasantly relieved when Susan made a joke to distract the team. Everyone laughed, and Bill was grateful that Susan had saved him.

Rev. Gene was the first to speak after the laughter subsided. "I wonder if we need to think about how our team is taking care of ourselves with all of these deaths? I know I have had some difficult days, trying to know how much grief I'm carrying around with me while I work."

Notice how each of the members of the hospice team respond to news of George's death. Susan's reaction, even her "saving" of Bill from embarrassment in the moment, is not unexpected, at least not by the team. She has a history of using humor to deflect the team's focus on feeling. That is, humor is one way Susan has of helping the team abide by the rule of Don't Feel.

Bill's reaction, we should say, is not indicative of a "direct" intersection of personal and team emotional process, but rather of the indirect but parallel process that more often occurs between team members and certain families.

Finally, we note that the team's spiritual caregiver responds in a way that blesses his own and everyone else's emotional process. We will want to return to what Rev. Gene has said in the final section of this chapter, to see in it as a response to the shame manifested by the presence of AEP. Rev. Gene gives us one example of how shame in team emotional process can be addressed and managed.

The important point to note is the overlay of multiple losses, including Bill's personal loss as a "carryover" from his own family. It is important to identify the pervasiveness of these losses and how some team members may be "positioned" to experience some patient losses to a greater extent than others.

Boundary Issues

AEP in the families that hospice teams serve presents temptations to team members that, when acted upon inappropriately, indicate the influence of AEP on TEP. One of these temptations is the perpetuation of relationships after the professional one has ended. Vulnerability to this can suggest AEP in one's own family. AEP raises issues related to uncertainties about belonging and individuation, and may be reflected in how one understands and acts on boundaries. As a result, often, transitions or endings can become problematic.

Susan called Wilma and arranged for a bereavement follow-up visit the next day. When she paid that visit, she found herself feeling sympathetic to Wilma. Wilma told her how much she had appreciated Susan's attention to her and George. She said that she felt they had George in common. Then Wilma asked Susan if she would come by to visit—regularly. "It would mean a lot to me if you'd stop by, maybe on your way home, once in a while," Wilma said. Susan looked at her and thought to herself, "She reminds me of my mother—but in a good way." To Wilma she said, "Sure. I'd enjoy that."

Figure 9.3 illustrates the way in which AEP can function in both the family and the team. Alliances or connections among and between specific members of the family and the team form "triangles"; these triangles suggest how team and family members may be in "alliance" or "dis-alliance" with particular family members. Here we see Susan's alliance with Wilma. We can see not only that it distinguishes her from the hospice team in general, but also that it distances Wilma from her own children, since she views Susan as more readily accessible in her grief over George.

Shame Awareness

At the intersection of the family's AEP and whatever level of AEP is influencing the team's emotional process, is this matter of shame—how shame is "bound" on the part of the family, and how shame is managed on the part of the team. What the AEP of the family brings to the emotional process of the team is awareness that along with anxiety, shame does need to be managed.

What we need to underscore here is that the AEP of the individual's family is likely *not* to be able to model well how to bind/manage shame. Thus the team, through its emotional process will need to grow both in its ability to become shame-aware, and in its ability to manage shame.

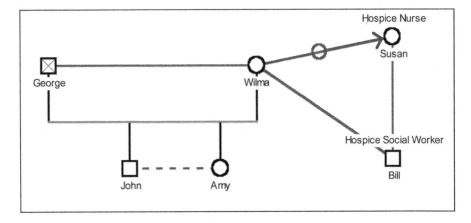

Figure 9.3 Addiction emotional process in the team: triangles.

Presuming that a team's emotional process can manage shame better than a family's, the team might then have a positive influence both on the AEP of its own members and on the addiction emotional processes of the families it serves.

Figure 9.4 illustrates the presence of shame for the team with respect to the Cinnamon family. The shading illustrates how the shame of addiction and death permeate the structures of both the team and the family. The influence of shame can be recognized as a dimension of the team's interaction, much as the influence of losses can be seen in both family and team members.

The following week at a team meeting, it was Jane's opportunity to present her bereavement plan of care. Jane offered her assessment: "We really need to think about how John, his ex-wife, Kate, and Amy are going to be helpful to foster Wilma's recovery while she is grieving. We will need to be more proactive than we have been." Susan was upset with Jane's reference to "recovery." "Wilma? You've got this all wrong. It's John who is the alcoholic. We probably need to help Wilma stay away from him!" But Jane replied that, in her case, Wilma's mourning and her beginning a process of recovery were linked. Thus supporting the one was also supporting the other.

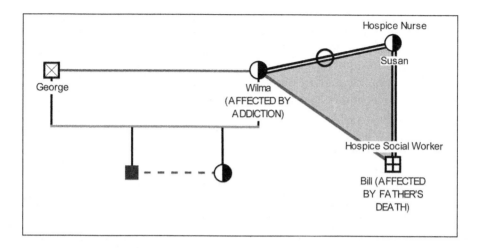

Figure 9.4 Shame and the team's emotional process.

SUMMARY: MANAGING SHAME
AND THE TEAM'S EMOTIONAL PROCESS

Throughout this chapter, we have stated the case for the necessity of the hospice team's emotional process not just to manage stress, but also to manage shame. We conclude this chapter by describing in general terms how shame management might address the influence and effects of addiction emotional process on team emotional process.

To begin we want to note that throughout this chapter, we have at least implied that shame management is a function of the entire hospice team. This is in contrast to stress management, which was discussed in the last chapter. In chapter 8 we stated that it is the responsibility of certain individuals on the team, typically the hospice manager, to be a "nonanxious presence," which then communicates calm to other members of the team. Stress management is a matter of individual, personal response.

In contrast to this, shame management is a matter of the response of the entire team. The entire team, as a system, in consensus, must recognize shame patterns, name them, and adjust accordingly. Shame management is a matter for TEP.

The reasons for this lie in the nature of "recovery" from AEP. As we illustrated in earlier chapters, "recovery" is necessitated not just on the part of the individual, identified addict, but also on the family as a whole. In addiction treatment, recovery is understood to turn not just on individual effort but upon belonging to supportive systems that provide acceptance and understanding.

Similarly, when AEP becomes manifest as an aspect of TEP, it is important that the *team* respond. Again, "recovery" is a process for the system, not merely the responsibility of any individual member of it.

Thus, if shame is originating in team members' replicating familial roles; or if the team finds that it has been living by certain "rules" that impede its coordination and cooperation; or if the team discovers that caring for particular families evokes in them responses that are attributable to AEP: Then the team becomes aware of the presence and influence of shame in its emotional process. Out of this awareness, it can strategize ways for managing the shame in its midst that are constructive for best practices in end-of-life care.

When the team accepts the presence of AEP, it can respond constructively and productively. It does not have to be ashamed of shame. It does not have to scapegoat individuals, exile them to their own personal recovery processes, pretend that shame is better handled privately, nor ignore the impact and significance of shame in its emotional process. Instead, it can realize that it is being challenged to provide for its own members a similar supportive environment of care around AEP that it would seek to provide to the patients and families on their census.

There are several benefits to TEP when it accepts the probable challenges of shame management. For one, team cohesion is enhanced. Belonging to the team becomes an affirmation of people belonging with each other. Levels of cooperation are deepened. The "we" of team transcends any "I" of its members.

Second, along these lines, an appreciation for collaboration and a willingness to collaborate replaces the mere sense of working together. When shame is being managed well, there is less apprehension and fear of being singled out. Thus, just as the interdisciplinary nature of hospice care is important to maintain, just as it takes a *team* to provide optimal service to someone who is dying and their family, so does it take a *collaborative* effort on the part of the team to address the influence of AEP. Effective *collaboration* among the interdisciplinary team depends on sharing, trusting, and appropriate boundary crossing, in order to meet the needs of patients and families (Payne, 2001; Taylor-See-hafer, 1998).

In this way, collaboration may be seen as a primary strategy for "recovery" on the team. Effective team collaboration is a way of addressing the disposition toward AEP that is likely to exist on the hospice team. The chronic shame that is likely to exist among hospice teams may become more acute when members of those teams are working with families where AEP is also present. This signals the need for teams to look more closely at shame and the recovery processes which promote collaborative team relationships based on mutual sharing, trusting, and feeling that supports professional caregiving.

Third, in this regard it would be beneficial for the hospice team to recognize itself as the "family" it often says it is or wants to be. If it were to do so, it might ask itself, how it might become a "healthy" family—a healthier family than most of those who have experienced AEP usually have. For this to happen, "recovery leadership" needs to become a shared task, a responsibility everyone takes on, because, after all, once the effects of AEP on TEP process are recognized, it becomes a matter of realizing that addiction affects how every one on the team functions, even as it affects the functioning of the team as a whole.

The aim, then, of "recovery leadership" and shame management in general is to enhance a *healthy* sense of family among the team. For what AEP brings forward is not only the realization that not all families are healthy, but also a quest, a hope for finding a healthy family—at least a healthier family, perhaps, than one has heretofore known. When TEP manages shame well, members of the team, in effect, become "re-familied." They become re-familiarized with the benefits of belonging. The results are healthier both for the members of the teams and for the families they are serving—and perhaps for the members of the families of the team members themselves.

Effective "recovery leadership" should ask itself how the hospice team might serve to develop mutually healing relationships, wherein caring for another brings about better caring for the self. If we are aware of relationships only when they are functioning to maintain certain aspects of emotional process, we may need to become more aware and more conscious that our patterns of thinking, feeling, and behaving have a functional purpose beyond their most immediate one. When that function is appropriately serving the purpose of end-of-life care, then it can also be personally healing for the hospice team members.

This is not to suggest that "healing oneself" should be the reason a hospice team member chooses to work in hospice. But it could well be a consequence. None of us grows alone, by ourselves. We all grow within systems that become healthier as their members become healthier. For hospice teams' emotional processes to become healthier, they will want to become aware of the presence of AEP. As they become aware of AEP they will want to address the ways that it arises within the team's emotional process. And, finally, the team will want to take steps in concert to differentiate what the presence of AEP means, both to the team itself and to the families they serve. The emotional processes of the hospice team will likely improve as members of the system learn to take at least these steps toward "recovery"—together, as the vocational "family" they already often see themselves to be.

REFERENCES

Baldisseri, M. (2007). Impaired health care professionals. *Critical Care Medicine,* *35*(2), 106–116.

Burke, R., & Fikrenbaum, L. (2009). Work motivations, work outcomes, and healthcare: Passion and addiction. *Journal of Business Ethics, 84*(2), 257–263.

Carnes, P. (2001). *Recovery zone: Making changes that last.* Carefree, AZ: Gentle Path Press.

Cicala, R. S. (2003). Substance abuse among physicians: What you need to know. *Hospital Physician, 39*(7), 39–46.

Dewees, M. (2006). *Contemporary social work practice.* Boston: McGraw-Hill.

Fletcher, C. C. (2001). Michigan's unique approach to treating impaired health care professionals. *Journal of Addictive Diseases, 20*(4), 101–116.

Fletcher, C. E., & Ronis, D .L. (2005). Satisfaction of impaired health care professionals with mandatory treatment and monitoring. *Journal of Addictive Diseases, 24,* 61–75.

Friedman, E. H. (1985) *Generation to generation: Family process in church and synagogue.* New York: Guilford Press.

Gallegos, K. V, Veit, F. W., Wilson, P. O., Porter, T., & Talbott, G. (1988). Substance abuse among health professionals. *Maryland Medical Journal, 37,* 191–197.

Harrington, A. (2006). The connection health care professionals make with dying patients. *Journal of Religion, Spirituality, and Aging, 18*(203), 169–173.

Hughes, P., Brandenburg, N., Baldwin, D., Storr, C., Williams, K., & Anthony, J. (1992). Prevalence of substance use among US physicians. *Journal of the American Medical Association, 267,* 2333–2339.

Jones, R. W. (2008). An impaired surgeon, a conflict of interest, and supervisory responsibilities. *Surgery, 135*(4), 449–451.

Al-Anon. (2002). *Opening our hearts, transforming our losses.* New York: Alcoholics Anonymous World Services.

Lambie, G. W., & Sias, S. M. (2007). Striving for meaningfulness and self acceptance. In Viers (Ed.), *The group therapist's notebook* (pp. 49–54). New York: Haworth Press.

Malleck, D. J. (2004). Professionalism and the boundaries of control. *Medical History, 48,* 175–198.

Martinez, R. (2002). The nature of illness experience: A course on boundaries. *Theoretical Medicine and Bioethics, 23*(3), 259–269.

Merlo, J. L., & Gold, M. S. (2008). Prescription opioid abuse and dependence among physicians: Hypotheses and treatment. *Harvard Review of Psychiatry, 16,* 181–194.

Payne, M. (2006). Team building: How, why and where? In P. Speck (Ed.), *Teamwork in palliative care: Fulfilling or frustrating* (pp. 117–136)? London: Oxford University Press.

Raistock, D., Russell, D., Tober, G., & Tindale, A. (2008). A survey of substance use by health care professionals. *Journal of Substance Use, 13*(1), 57–69.

Substance Abuse and Mental Health Services Administration. (2002). *Results from the 2001 Household Survey on Drug Abuse, Volume I: Summary of national findings* (NHSDA Series H-17, DHHS Publication No. SMA 02-3758). Rockville, MD: Author.

Substance Abuse and Mental Health Services Administration. (2007). *DASIS report June 28, 2007: Admissions. Substance Abuse and Mental Health Services Administration short reports.* Washington, DC: Author.

Talbott, G. D., & Martin, M. (1991). Impaired healthcare professionals. *Critical Care Medicine, 19*(2), S.106–116.

Taylor-Seehafer, M. (1998). Nurse–physician collaboration. *Journal of the American Academy of Nurse Practitioners, 10*(9), 387–391.

Thornburg, P.I., Schim, S., Paige, V., & Grubaugh, K. (2008). Nurses' experience of caring while letting go. *Journal of Hospice and Palliative Care Nursing, 10*(6), 382–391.

Trinkoff, A., & Storr, C. (1998). Substance use among nurses: Differences between specialties. *American Journal of Public Health, 88,* 581–585.

White, W., & McClelland, T. (2008). Addiction as a chronic disorder. *Journal of Substance Abuse Treatment, 35*(1), 1–12.

Whitehead, J. D., & Whitehead, E. (1995) *Shadows of the heart: A spirituality of the negative emotions.* New York: Crossroads.

10 The Spiritual Care of Addiction and Dying

The night that Wilma woke him to ask whether he loved her had already been a fitful one for George. Funny, he had been thinking the same thing: Why had he married her? Why hadn't he married another woman? He'd had the chance. Why had he gotten so comfortable so quickly, in the marriage? That was when Wilma woke him. Bad timing.

When he rolled over and faced the wall, he couldn't go back to sleep. It seemed he had all of these questions: Why had he stayed in the same job? Why hadn't he taken that promotion? Then he began wondering about his children: Why did Amy treat him like she did, with suspicion and distance? Why did John become an alcoholic? And why did he insist he was much healthier now? George wondered whether his children thought he was a good father.

Then he realized why he had snapped at Wilma. It wasn't just because he had been wondering at the time whether he really did love her. It was because he had wanted more than anything to hear her say that she loved him.

From the outset, our goal has been to advocate for considering the family as the unit of care, both in end-of-life care and in addiction treatment. To accomplish this, we have emphasized the importance of our *relationships*, especially those we share as families. It has been our hope that by better understanding ourselves in the context of our families, we might provide better treatment and care for persons with addictions, and, certainly, for persons at the end of their lives. For "patients" do not die; people do. Thus addicts need to be restored to a sense of their own personhood, just as much as they need treatment for their disease. At the end of our lives and in the course of our addictions, what is essentially at stake is our humanity: Both experiences are opportunities to be confirmed in the significance of our being human.

We understand the benefits of the medical model for both end-of-life care and addiction treatment. There are medical aspects to both life events that need to be identified and acted upon. Similarly, the business model for conducting health care is also important. We understand and appreciate the interface between the practice of medicine and business, and we offer here no critique of that.

Rather, we are attempting to articulate a more *holistic* understanding of the person receiving end-of-life care that preserves his/her personhood and humanity. To that end, we have proposed a form of family emotional process (FEP) that we refer to as *addiction emotional process* (AEP). We hope we have sufficiently identified the differences between these processes, and made a case for understanding AEP as its own familial phenomenon.

We believe that what AEP reveals is the significant role of shame. Through AEP we are able to see how shame functions in relationships among family members and that shame becomes acute in the process of dying and grieving.

Others have speculated about shame as an internalized "master emotion," and its relationship to a wide range of social and cultural issues such as self-esteem/concept issues, depression, addiction, eating disorders, bullying, suicide, family violence, and sexual assault (Bradshaw, 1988; Brown, 2003; Scheff, 2003). Our point is that shame is not merely an emotion we experience individually. Instead, the way shame is defined and functions points directly to the *relational* context of shame. Shame is experienced in relationships.

Shame is linked to our longing to belong; it "names the inner attunement we bring to our encounters with other people" (Whitehead & Whitehead, 1985, p. 103). As Brown (2003) defines it, shame is "an intensely painful feeling or experience of believing we are flawed, and therefore unworthy of acceptance and belonging" (p. 45).

Understanding the role that shame plays in families with AEP helps us to understand our personal experience of shame in a way that does not further pathologize or condemn us. In other words, to feel shame is not in itself our *fault*. On the contrary, it is an affirmation of our humanity. The ways that we experience shame—or deny that we are experiencing shame—can be attributed to how we learned to manage shame through the emotional processes of our families.

This becomes especially important as we come to the end of our lives, for the journey through our final days is often one replete with shame experiences, including the stigma of dying and grieving. The role that shame plays during the dying and grieving processes, as people struggle to understand the *meaning* of their lives, is our focus here. This meaning-making is essential to dying and grieving, and shame awareness is integral to the meanings that are made. Whether or not one can come to a sense that one has lived a meaningful life, often depends on how one manages shame—both in the course of dying or grieving, and in the course of *reflecting* on one's life—thinking about what occurred and how one's time was spent.

This meaning-making is essentially a *spiritual* process, both for the individual and the family. As we said in chapter 1, from a family systems point of view, a death in the family is less a personal experience than an event in the life or the history of the family. Thus what is important, spiritually speaking, is the meaning that family members take from the event. That meaning will speak to their sense of themselves as a family, and give hospice professionals a sense of how they will grieve. In this chapter we will see how end-of-life professionals might participate in the spiritual processes involved as the family, as a whole, through its individual members, articulates what their life together has meant to them, and manages their shame in the process.

To understand how hospice professionals can bring appropriate spiritual care to families in this transition, it will be helpful to understand more about how shame functions in both its healthy and its toxic forms; to understand why shame necessitates expressly *spiritual* care, even if it has psychosocial aspects; and to learn how addressing shame in appropriately caring ways brings about a greater level of health in a family, as well as the individual members of it.

TOXIC AND HEALTHY SHAME

As a human experience central to our experience of ourselves in relationships, shame is remarkable both for its universality and for its variety. In chapter 5, we said that adequately understanding shame required taking into account three interactive layers of human experience: Our culture or society; our families; and our individual selves. We can see these three "concentric circles" influencing each other in nearly every study of shame we have examined.

Although shame is often seen as a cause of emotional distress (Brown, 2003), there is evidence that a healthy sense of shame is possible, and indeed is important to our personal functioning. *A healthy sense of shame promotes our appropriately protected and positive experiences of others.* James and Evelyn Whitehead, for example, make this claim: "With proper care, a positive sense of shame matures into a resident strength in us—a virtue" (Whitehead & Whitehead, 1995, p. 111). Among the virtues they name as based in a positive sense of shame are humility, dignity, and chastity. Humility alerts "us to the limits of our strength and gifts" (p. 112). Dignity has to do with "an enduring sense of our worth" (p. 112). And chastity is "an inner sense of modesty that protects us as we attempt both to reveal and conceal ourselves" (p. 113). Properly understood, humility, dignity, and, as we will choose to put it, *modesty* are all significant aspects of our experience of ourselves at the end of our lives. Moreover, brought properly to bear, these three virtues become aspects of how spiritual care can enhance our familial relationships, adding a depth of meaning to our life's final chapter.

For us, the key in the Whiteheads' writing is the word "matures." We are capable of experiencing shame differently throughout the course of life. How we are responded to by others can damage the way shame functions in us. "The healthy response of shame, bruised this early, turns toxic" (Whitehead & Whitehead, 1995, p. 96). Bradshaw (1988), who speaks of shame as a "state of being," describes how this happens in psychodynamic terms:

> When healthy shame is transformed into toxic shame, it is called the 'internalization process.' The healthy feeling of shame is lost, and a frozen state of being emerges, whereby a person believes himself to be flawed and defective as a human being. (p. 23)

Once toxic, our experience of shame can change. We can be "healed" of shame's toxicity (Bradshaw, 1988). Shame might become healthy for us again. This is what we believe the Whiteheads meant when they said that shame "matures."

According to Erik Erikson, shame arises, along with doubt, in the course of our coming to a sense of our autonomy, which entails mastering the "social modalities of holding on and letting go" (Erikson, 1963, p. 251). Our environment must also *protect* us against "meaningless and arbitrary experiences of shame and of early doubt" (p. 252). Whether or not and how this protection is provided is itself an aspect of our shame experience. "Shame supposes that one is completely exposed and conscious of being looked at: in one word, self-conscious. One is visible and not ready to be visible" (p. 252).

Several aspects of what Erikson is saying here are instructive for us. The first is the notion that shame is related to our autonomy, because it is precisely this sense of ourselves as autonomous that is challenged and compromised in the course of our dying. Maintaining patient autonomy is one of the goals of hospice care.

Second, that shame is related to our "holding onto and letting go" relates directly to our mourning. Through grief, we struggle with the balancing of how to hold onto our loved ones, and how to let them go. It is no wonder that shame would be experienced as an aspect of grief, as well as of end-of-life care.

Third, Erikson (1963) makes it clear that we experience shame in the interaction with and through the regard of others. Shame here, even in a developmental psychological sense, has to do with how our "environment" behaves toward us—whether it "protects" us or not—and how we *feel* about being seen—and our awareness that we are not alone, but are being looked at and scrutinized. Even in Erikson's developmental sense of shame, relationships with others are essential.

The interpersonal nature of our being, growth, and development is shaped and affected by the societies in which we live. The perspective we have articulated here is congruent with this. We take our focus to be on the family, as a system, to highlight our human inter-relatedness. Maintaining this point of view, we argue, is central to adequate and especially excellent end-of-life care. Second, it is particularly during our dying, but also during our grieving, that our toxic or "negative" experience of shame is available for healing, or at least alteration. It is because these are transitional experiences, when we are, perhaps, at our most vulnerable, that our shame might most "mature."

At a time in our lives when shame and shame-related issues are many and open, it is important for us to make the following affirmation: *If shame (particularly painful experiences of shame) entered our lives through our relationships, then it is through relationships that the pain of shame might be relieved.* If we are to have a positive experience of shame, then this *transformation* must occur in the experience of ourselves and others in relationships. As we will see, virtue can be nurtured in us *by* virtue. That is, by being in a relationship with those who have matured a positive sense of shame in themselves, we can mature a positive sense of shame in ourselves.

This is why *systems* are so important to our shame experience. Systems of relationships can both contribute to our experience of shame as toxic and painful—and can be the means for relief. Our participation in systems that have a positive sense of the place of shame in the human experience is palliative, if not completely healing. Such systems could be called "virtuous" in themselves, and we believe that hospice sets out, in a spiritual sense, to be a "virtuous" system for end-of-life care.

DISTINGUISHING SHAME AND GUILT

Being able to distinguish between shame and guilt becomes essential, significant, and important in both end-of-life care and in addiction treatment.

Erikson suggests that our confusion about shame and guilt is somewhat sociocultural. Even though we commonly seem to prefer guilt to shame, and thus speak of it more easily, shame precedes guilt. "If guilt concerns what we have done, shame concerns who we are. Guilt addresses correctness, but shame addresses worth" (Whitehead & Whitehead, 1995, p. 111). We have employed these definitions in service of a family systems perspective in order to emphasize the roles of shame and guilt in AEP. We accounted for the role of blame in transmuting shame into guilt in AEP. Understanding this role of blame not only underscores one source of the pain of addiction, but it also reveals how difficult it is in AEP to separate our actions as faulty from our sense of ourselves as faulty. This is why being able to separate shame and guilt is pivotal to addiction treatment and recovery.

The research of Dearing, Stuewig, and Tangney (2005), for example, positively correlates "shame-proneness" with alcohol and drug addiction, and shows that "guilt-proneness" was negatively correlated. Although it is the case that "addiction and shame are inseparable" (Fossum & Mason, 1986), *focusing* on shame was shown to be not likely to produce positive therapeutic results (Dearing, Steuwig, & Tangney, 2005). Granted, the pain of shame is debilitating because it affects one's core sense of self and leaves shame-prone individuals vulnerable to a variety of emotional problems. However, because "the focus of shame is on the defective self, this painful emotion also has the effect of impairing empathy, which can result in a host of interpersonal difficulties" (Dearing et al., 2005). In other words, because shame *impairs* an addict's empathic capacity, focusing on shame and shame-proneness was not in itself therapeutically beneficial.

Instead, distinguishing guilt from shame did have some positive therapeutic benefits. Even though guilt, too, is painful, the feelings of guilt "are less disabling than shame and are likely to motivate the individual in a positive direction toward reparation or change" (Dearing et al., 2005, p. 1401). Thus, "shame-free guilt is positively correlated with adaptive characteristics, such as empathy" (Dearing et al., 2005, p. 1400).

Perhaps concentrating therapeutic focus on guilt as opposed to shame *works* because actions are more concrete and demonstrable than are internal senses of oneself. Actions and their consequences can be pointed out and responsibility can be chosen. "Guilt-prone individuals are inclined to take responsibility for their actions," rather than blame others, "because feelings of guilt often lead to attempts at reparation and atonement; guilt-proneness helps to foster healthy interpersonal relationships" (Dearing et al., 2005, p. 1394). When guilt is accepted, matters can be rectified and relationships can be mended. We agree that distinguishing between guilt and shame would be useful, and not only in treating problems of addiction, but also in providing excellent end-of-life care.

The third reason for distinguishing shame and guilt is not just to suggest that health and recovery might be aided by shifting "maladaptive shame reactions to more adaptive guilt responses" (Dearing et al., 2005, p. 1394), but also to recognize that the experience of shame might be so painful, that shame in itself gives rise to certain "maladaptive shame responses." For instance, many might wonder: If shame is so common and so central to the experience of being human, how does it come to be that so many people seem to behave shamelessly, as if shame did not matter to them? By all appearances, some people are shame impaired. How do we account for that?

We believe that AEP tells us a great deal about shame, about how it is experienced through one's participation in a family system. We not only receive our shame training and shame conditioning in our families, but we also receive from our families a sense of what to *do* with our shame—how to behave when we feel shame. One way to behave when we feel ashamed is to *deny* what we are feeling. The denial of shame (or shamelessness) can result in a sense of becoming *numbed* to shame. Thus, the shame *in* AEP is precisely what leads to the shame-lessness *of* AEP.

We could say that it is possible to become "shame overloaded." Erikson (1963) wrote that "too much shaming does not lead to genuine propriety but to a secret determination to try to get away with things, unseen—if, indeed, it does not result in defiant shamelessness" (p. 253). When others respond in shaming ways to shame we already feel, not only is an opportunity to learn "virtue" lost, but in order to protect *ourselves* from the pain of feeling unworthy and deeply flawed, we numb, verbally deny, and behave as if shame did not matter.

The denial of shame, and consequent shameless behaviors, does not mean that shame is not experienced. In fact, it might indicate high levels of unhealthy or toxic shame. If addiction is one means of binding anxiety in a family, but at the same time has the effect of releasing shame that then must be bound, then perhaps the identified addict in the family is not the least, but the *most,* shame-sensitive person in the family—in Dearing's terms, the most "shame-prone." Bradshaw (1988) confirms this when he writes: "Neurotic shame is the root and fuel of all compulsive/addictive behaviors" (p. 15).

What are end-of-life professionals to *do* about the shame and guilt that their patients and families are experiencing? Can shame be "detoxi-fied"? Can shame come to take an appropriate and constructive place in a person's life—especially if that person is dying?

The answer depends on end-of-life professionals being able to distinguish between guilt and shame, for each requires its own response from those providing end-of-life care. In a word, guilt and shame require different *spiritual* responses.

For those in AEP, it helps to learn that not every faulty act, not every mistake, is a reflection of a faulty self—even if that is what those in AEP most fear. One step in the maturation process of shame is for people to be able to say, "I *did* wrong," and for that admission to be a confirmation of themselves as persons. Admitting guilt without blame transmuting that guilt into a sense of being unworthy is a step forward in self-differentiation and growth.

The difficulty for families in AEP, and why the lines between shame and guilt tend to get blurred as they do, has to do with the lowered level of self-differentiation in such families. It takes a rather well-differentiated parent to teach a child how to treat their own shame constructively. Less well-differentiated parents are more likely to add shame by shaming. When shaming is used abusively, it turns toxic. This is also how shame becomes chronic, and is "passed down" through the generations. One must be taught how to handle shame in a way that promotes self-protection, does not "recruit" fear and anger "to speak for it" (Whitehead & Whitehead, 1995, p. 98), and connects a healthy sense of shame to a virtuous sense of self. For those in AEP, this lesson is not likely to occur.

ADDRESSING SHAME AND GUILT CONSTRUCTIVELY

Accepting that shame itself is not likely to be "healed" is to ratify that shame is chronic. Although the toxicity of shame might be mitigated, the wounds remain. The shame that is universal in the human condition and chronic in human relationships such as the family cannot be eliminated. Rather, one's shame can be experienced differently—constructively, positively. The shame that we carry in ourselves and in our families can *mature*. It matures as we improve our self-differentiation. The place of shame in our emotional processes improves, along the lines of recovery.

In family systems terms, being able to separate shame and guilt is itself a process of self-differentiation. A more whole, and complete self emerges: I am *guilty* perhaps of doing something wrong; however, just because I did something wrong does not mean that I am wrong or that there is something "wrong" with me.

As we separate guilt and shame, we begin to realize that they deserve different responses—from within ourselves, and from others. Both guilt and shame are indications of ruptures in our relationships. Admitting guild releases it from blame's attempt to bind shame, and results in a step forward in self-differentration and growth. Shame, however, cannot be addressed with forgiveness.

The reason for this lies in the difference between acting and being. One can be forgiven for one's actions—hence forgiveness is an antidote for guilt. There are processes for forgiveness: Confession, making amends, asking for forgiveness, and (perhaps) receiving it. In spiritual terms, one can atone for one's guilt.

But as for shame—a sense of one's own faultiness—no forgiveness is needed! How can one be forgiven for who one is? This is not possible. But *thinking* that forgiveness is somehow needed or required is evidence of the confusion between shame and guilt.

Instead of forgiveness, what is required as an antidote for toxic or painful shame is *acceptance*. Morrison (2003) explains, "whereas guilt motivates the patient to confess, shame motivates one to conceal." That is why while "for guilt, the antidote is forgiveness; for shame, it is the healing response of acceptance of the self, despite its weakness, defects, and failures" (Morrison, 2003, p. 82). A clue to the acceptance that shame-mitigation and shame-maturation requires can be found in The Serenity Prayer: *God, grant me the serenity to accept the things I cannot change; the courage to change the things I can; and the wisdom to know the difference.* For our purposes, this prayer articulates the wisdom to separate guilt from shame; the courage to mend the damages stemming from the actions for which we are guilty; and the serenity of acceptance of who we are: flawed, but not worthless, as we, in self-rejection, might otherwise conclude.

Using a prayer to illustrate a constructive way of addressing shame and guilt exemplifies why guilt and shame call for *spiritual* care. The forgiveness processes that address guilt can be spiritual in nature. And the acceptance experiences that address and mitigate our shame are likewise spiritual in nature.

We might more readily understand how and why spiritual care becomes important here if we appreciate the magnitude of shame which exceeds its comprehension by narrow, even multidisciplinary, points of view. Shame is "something that could not be considered exclusively psychological, social, or cultural" (Brown, 2003, p. 45). In its ubiquity and universality, shame *transcends* these academic constructs. Speaking of shame in spiritual terms thus becomes one way of grasping its transcendent universality.

Not only is there validity in taking a spiritual approach to understanding shame, but there is also validity in taking a *spiritual practice* toward shame. As we will see, this spiritual practice is less a matter of individual devotion or personal dedication, than it is a matter of our discovering in and through relationships our *acceptability*. It is not for each of us to *heal* ourselves the wounds of shame, but rather to *meet* each other in our mutual and common shame-woundedness, and thereby find relief and palliation from the pain of shame that each of us experiences in our own way.

To comprehend how the toxicity of shame can be mitigated and shame can be matured, we need to shift our perspective from the psychological understandings of family systems theory toward the *spirituality* of relationships. This is in keeping with our focus on providing excellent care to the dying and their families because *end-of-life care is essentially spiritual care.* Dying and facing death (one's own and/or that of a family member), and the grieving that occurs in these processes, are *spiritual* as well as medical, social, and psychological processes.

Earlier in the book, we defined the "spiritual" as that which concerns itself with *meanings*, especially the concern for ultimate meanings that arise at the end of life. This is why end-of-life care is spiritual care: The language of spirituality best captures these ultimate meanings; its perspectives frame human experience in ways that matter such as in the understanding of shame. Taking a spiritual perspective in end-of-life care means focusing on the *meaning* of how and why family systems and their members function in the ways that they do.

To frame our spiritual approach to end-of-life caring, we will draw from the three spiritual aspects or consequences of addiction that we named in chapter 3: idolatry, isolation, and intimacy challenges, as these are expressed by the family as a system. We will discuss each from an individual's sense of meaning, yet remain committed to a perspective that comprehends each person within the family system. Although the family functions as a system, the participants in the system draw their own spiritual meanings or significances for themselves from that participation.

Viewing the family system and its individual members in this kind of alternating foreground/background perspective is our way of doing justice to the spiritual meaning of the relationships one has—or has had—in one's family.

WHY ADDRESSING SHAME IS IMPORTANT IN END-OF-LIFE CARE

The end of our lives is the juncture of our most dreaded experiences, all of which have their shame-releasing aspects to them:

> The dynamics of this final stage of the life cycle and the dramatic dependency of the dying upon their helpers reveal the fallacy of the cultural conceit that thinks of self-realization as an individual achievement....The sense of shame exercised *by others* is an intrinsic component in the ability of the dying to live out the final days in a manner compatible with their self-image. (Schneider, 1992, p. 80, emphasis added)

These "others" include not just our immediate family members. They also include the situations and institutions of care in which we are likely to find ourselves when we are dying. For instance, Schneider notes that since many die in hospitals or nursing homes, intrusions into our privacy are unavoidable: "We are forced to undergo this most private experience of life in a thoroughly public setting. For many, the only protection is the collective sense of shame and discretion exercised in relation to a dying person...." (Schneider, 1992, p. 80). To some degree, hospice (especially home hospice) mitigates this sense of public intrusion into our most private time. In that way, home hospice, simply in its structure, addresses at least some of our end-of-life shame issues.

Yet hospice is an extension of our medical care system, and there are some who see our health care system itself as shame-based. Expressing his frustration over not getting appropriate care for one of his patients, Wheeler (2003) wrote: "no resources were available under a health care system that is itself founded on shame (if you are poor, you fall outside the net of belongingness and care, including health care; this exclusion is the very definition of shame)" (p. 221). The business of health care, speaking in the language of "affordability" and "economic feasibility," may be unaware of its shame-related aspects and consequences.

We may be ashamed of ourselves simply because we are dying! Schneider quotes Robert Neale, in his classic, *The Art of Dying*, as follows: "Some of us are ashamed to participate in dying. We die in a hospital....To be in bed is embarrassing....There may be a bed-pan or medical paraphernalia connected with the body—that is, there are certain intimate doings with the body which are not thought fit for the public eye" (Schneider, 1992, p. 81). And not just the public *eye*. Dying brings with it many odors, for which the dying themselves often feel compelled to apologize. The disintegration of our bodies, and the failures and limitations of our wills as we die contribute to a rather constant sense of shame unfolding for us.

Our individual experiences of dying have in them some common threads, all of which are aspects of the tapestry we have made of our experiences of shame throughout our lives. Vulnerability is one. Our vulnerability leads us to feel exposed—and helpless to cover ourselves. (This is true not only for our experiences of dying, but also of illness. In some ways, periods of being ill prepare us for the indignities and exposures that often attend dying.)

In addition, our vulnerability and our helplessness can elicit an embarrassing sense of regression. In childhood, shame came when we struggled with the eliminative functions of our bodies (Erikson, 1963). These issues of control rise again, anew, for us as adults when we lose these early learned masteries.

As we die, whatever psychological, sociological, and cultural constructs we used for managing our shame become increasingly ineffective. "In dying, an individual often must live out a diminished humanity....We are repeatedly faced with situations that remind us of our inability to live up to our ego-ideal—the situation which, in analytic language, is the basis for shame" (Schneider, 1992, p. 80).

In many cases, the process of dying is itself a defining moment of shame. We are seen when we do not want to be and are not ready to be. We are pained by our exposure and from that, by our sense of feeling worthless. We want to hide; to disappear; to be invisible. In fact, our dying can be a literal realization of what we had previously taken only metaphorically. When ashamed, we probably said something to the effect of, "I could have died!" What we may have taken most from our lifelong experiences of shame is a kind of mortification. This connection in our language speaks to something felt, and realized in the process of dying: "Shame is experienced as a wish to die; dying, especially in our society, is shameful" (Schneider, 1992, p. 79).

Shame is not merely an *individual* experience of personal exposure, helplessness, and vulnerability, but one witnessed by and participated in by one's caregivers. It is not enough to think that what occurs for the individual as she or he dies happens only among strangers (however, that might be true in institutional medical settings). Rather, from our perspective, we die as we lived: Among family, whether that be because they are literally present, or because we have internalized them, and we take them with us unto death.

This is one reason why, for all we may otherwise understand about shame as a personal experience, in end-of-life care shame arises among families providing care. Above, and especially in chapters 6 and 7, we discussed the variety of ways that shame arises in caregiving, caretaking, and grieving. Shame arises in visceral and immediate ways for family members. They may remark, for instance, to hospice professionals that they had "never seen" their family member like this—and hadn't wanted to!

One of the big challenges for end-of-life care professionals is: How are they to approach and behave in a situation so rife with shame, yet be able to preserve or enhance what positive sense of shame might be possible and certainly keep the situational shame from becoming toxic? That is to say, end-of-life professionals are aware of the likely prevalence of certain shame issues that can present with almost every patient and family. As the "cultural conceits" with which the individual and the family have lived begin to erode and vanish, how end-of-life care professionals respond to the shame will make a significant difference in how the dying person and their family experience—and remember—this time, and each other.

End-of-life professionals can reflect a positive sense of shame by considering the three virtues that the Whiteheads named earlier: Humility, dignity, and modesty. How can they promote humility in circumstances that can be humiliating? What can they do to preserve everyone's dignity, at a time when the patient and family members are not likely to be able to preserve their own dignity themselves? And how can they best address the modesty-challenges of end-of-life care? Managing positively the acute shame experienced in families during dying and grief in just these three areas alone will have a significantly positive impact on the emotional process of that family.

For end-of-life professionals, having a positive sense of shame means that *they are not ashamed of shame*; they do not shrink from shame when they see it. They are willing to engage with shame and to promote a positive sense of shame in end-of-life care. It is important for us to remember that, when it functions at its best, shame is meant to "pre-serve" our personhood and the meaningfulness of our lives. Shame is meant to keep us from being "devalued," from becoming mere bodies to be counted. "Shame functions as a protective covering against this stripping-bare of the individual" (Schneider, 1992, p. 78).

Unfortunately, many of us are less accepting of our own shame, less comfortable with our shame, and less confident that shame can be experienced in a constructive way. This is because we have not often had a positive experience of shame. The irony is that many who have had negative experiences of shame find themselves seeking precisely the professions that are likely to be providing end-of-life care, as we discussed in chapter 9.

It is fitting that in end-of-life care, people who are dying and griev-ing, thus those for whom "shame immersion" is most new and unset-tling, come to meet hospice professionals who are shame-aware and have found the wisdom of becoming shame-mature so that they might be of better service to those for whom they care.

SPIRITUAL CARE AND SHAME AT THE END OF LIFE

Issues of shame, shame management, and shame experience abound in end-of-life care—in the patient, among the family, and within and among the health professionals who provide end-of-life care. Moreover, shame is ubiquitous regardless of the particular emotional process of the family. All families, not just those in AEP, concern themselves with shame. However, by using families with AEP as an example, we can better understand what all families need from end-of-life care.

Knowing that shame is so significant at the end of life, we consider the three spiritual aspects of addiction—idolatry, isolation, and intimacy issues—and illustrate how hospice professionals, in the course of their spiritual care of their patients and their patients' families, can address the shame and the shame-related issues that arise. As we will see, addressing each of the three spiritual aspects of addiction calls for its

Exhibit 10.1

Spritual Responses to Shame

When the spiritual aspect is:	the spiritual response is to be:	calling for the virtue of:
Idolatry	Mutuality	Humility
Isolation	Community	Dignity
Intimacy impairment	Compassion	Modesty

own response and an aim to develop a particular virtue. The correspondence we will develop is depicted in Exhibit 10.1.

By stressing spiritual care, we mean to comment both on the limitations of psychosocial care in addressing shame, and to discourage end-of-life care professionals from taking a strictly therapeutic or treatment approach to it. It would be misguided for end-of-life professionals to think only psychotherapeutically about the shame their patients and families are experiencing. Rather, a spiritual approach can be more constructive. The aim is less the "healing" of chronic shame than its transformation from a negative to a positive. Again, this is in keeping with the hospice aim of care rather than cure.

Even so, we want to respect the fact that one's shame, and one's family's shame, is difficult to talk about. Brené Brown (2003), in formulating what she calls "Shame Resilience Theory," says that one of the four components of being shame resilient is the ability to "speak shame," to "possess the language and emotional competence to discuss and deconstruct shame" (Brown, 2003, p. 48). Because putting one's sense of shame into words and identifying the *meaning* of one's experience of shame is not a skill at which many are adept, end-of-life professionals may find that teaching this skill is how they can best care for their patients and their families. Such pedagogy is itself a spiritual enterprise.

The Spiritual Care of the Shame of Idolatry

In providing spiritual care to families with addiction histories, hospice professionals are likely to notice the effects that addiction has had on the family's emotional process. They are likely to be less adept at making the spiritual assessment of "*idolatry.*" But if we remember that addiction entails a primary attachment to an object, we can understand that this is an appropriate assessment, in spiritual terms.

The chronic shame that has originated in this attachment can be addressed by establishing relationships with family members based on *mutuality.* Mutuality is "the awareness that life's most precious realities—love, wisdom, sobriety—are attained only in the giving of them and are given only in the openness to receive them" (Kurtz & Ketcham, 1992, p. 85).

Mutuality in end-of-life spiritual care entails a willingness on the part of the end-of-life professional to be *vulnerable.* Vulnerability does not mean disclosing personal information about oneself nor being inappropriately personal. But it does mean recognizing the great (and likely one-sided) vulnerability of the patient and the family. In offering a degree of mutuality, the end-of-life professional meets the family's great vulnerability with a portion of his or her own, in order that a *mutual* relationship might be formed.

This mutual relationship alters the object-oriented relationship of idolatry in addiction by restoring a person-to-person connection. To affect mutuality in AEP means that shame is likely to be experienced, and judgment feared. This is why it is important that the end-of-life professional practice the virtue of *humility.* In recognizing and appreciating one's limitations and in demonstrating a degree of acceptance, both of oneself and of the one being cared for, the health-care professional can transform the malfunctioning shame of idolatry, mitigate the degree of humiliation, and offer to the person of care an acceptance that is affirming.

Bill, the social worker from Heart of Gold Hospice, finally reached John by phone. Bill explained who he was, and expressed regret that, in all the weeks John's father had been on hospice, they'd never met.

At first John was defensive, saying that he seldom got to his parents' house, but then he mentioned that in fact he'd been able to get over there more than he had before.

Something in John's voice led Bill to say, "I hope you don't mind, but I have a personal question to ask." John nervously agreed. "Have you and your Dad talked? I mean," Bill said, *"about his being your father and your being his son?"*

John was quiet, and Bill worried whether he'd overstepped. After all, it was their first conversation. But then John said, "You know, I've been meaning to." Bill suggested that John have that conversation with his father soon. "Your Dad's time is short," Bill said, "and I just think you'd regret it more if you didn't."

The Spiritual Care of the Shame of Isolation

A spiritual assessment of a family in AEP is likely to include notice of the emotional *isolation* through which the chronic shame has been bound. Perhaps family members have become so adept at creating isolating situations and alliances that hospice team members feel pitted against one another, "split," with some team members described as acceptable and positive, and others rejected and or found to be unacceptable.

The spiritual care approach that best addresses isolation is one that embraces *community*. By this we mean, in the most basic way, a sense of teamwork. Spiritual care is provided in concert, with a sense of co-ordination.

But we also mean an implicit (and sometimes explicit) invitation to meet with family members together. The dying are often isolated, and it is all too easy for hospice professionals to focus on family members who are verbal, or who can dialogue. By creating a sense of community for the entire family, the hospice professional affirms the virtue of *dignity*, not just as a personal quality, but as an aspect of ourselves that we depend on others to preserve when we cannot. The hospice professional treats all the members of the family with dignity—and guards against dynamics in the family's emotional process that would be shaming. By including the dying person in the family's life, thus modeling ways in which no one in the family feels isolated from one another, the hospice professional provides an opportunity for the chronic shame that had been bound in isolation to be transformed into a positive experience—with each one in the family respecting the other's inherent dignity. This is likely to create a new and positive experience of belonging for that family.

In all of the time that the Cinnamon family had been on hospice, Bill and Susan had not paid another joint visit since the first one, when George was admitted. At a team meeting, Bill said that he thought George and Wilma were spending a lot of time alone, each in their own parts of the house. Susan said that every time she went, she examined George, and then went to the living room to talk with Wilma. Susan and Bill decided another joint visit was in order.

They arrived together, and Bill stayed with Wilma while Susan examined George. When she was done, Bill said to Wilma, "C'mon. Let's take some chairs in and the three of us will sit with George for a while." Wilma was surprised, but compliant. Susan made George as comfortable as possible, sitting up in his hospital bed. And the other three of them formed a kind of semi-circle around his side rail. To all appearances, they didn't seem to talk about anything in particular; they were just talking. But then, something Wilma said prompted George to say, "Remember that time we went to the lake, just the two of us, when the kids were still young? I think that was just about the best weekend we'd had in a long time!" Wilma said, "Yes. That was pretty romantic...." This reminiscence led to another, and for a little while anyway, it seemed to Susan and Bill that George and Wilma were actually enjoying themselves.

The Spiritual Care of the Shame of Intimacy Impairment

The hospice professional who assesses the AEP of a family will likely note, in spiritual terms, the ways that family members are *intimacy impaired*. Spiritually speaking, this is how they have managed the chronic shame of their belonging—by not letting other people get genuinely close. Likely, in the way that family members speak with each other, the hospice professional will notice a tendency to blame, and see it for what it is: A means for transmuting shame into guilt.

In providing spiritual care with such families, *compassion* is needed. Compassion is an ability to take the pain or suffering of another onto oneself, and to hold it there for a time—and then to release it, so that another's suffering does not become one's own.

In offering compassion to families experiencing the release of shame, the hospice professional practices the virtue of *modesty*, that is to say, to be comfortable with one's own abilities to protect oneself, without withdrawing or diminishing one's affections and connections with others. The hospice professional thus models "a skillful confidence in the dance of human interaction" (Whitehead & Whitehead, 1995, p. 114) that encourages family members to develop in themselves a different, positive sense of shame, one that allows for a higher degree of comfort in belonging. Families whose shame is transformed in this way will find they are better able to comfort each other in their mourning. They will increase their ability and desire to trust each other.

Bill arrived at the Cinnamon home at a time when Wilma had gone to the store, and Amy was taking care of her father. George was asleep, so Bill and Amy had a conversation in the living room.

Bill simply asked how things were going for her. Seeing Amy hesitate before answering, he added, "I mean, how are you managing looking after both your father and mother and your own family?" Amy looked him square in the eye, and said, "By the help and strength of God." Bill tried not to be too taken aback. He said, "I gather your faith means a lot to you." Amy agreed that her faith did mean a lot to her, and relaxing just a little, she told Bill that reading daily devotionals every morning and the Bible every night before she went to sleep was how she "did it." Bill, realizing that in her own way, Amy was telling him something very personal about herself, thanked her for what she'd said, and told her that he was glad that she had this refuge and solace during this difficult time. Something in the way Bill spoke told Amy he was sincere. She liked that he used the words "refuge and solace." That felt right.

Becoming Spiritual Caregivers

Even though there may be a professional spiritual caregiver on the hospice team, it is appropriate for every professional to develop his/her own spiritual capacities, as well as his/her ability to provide spiritual care. And since shame at the end of life is a universal, or near universal experience, it behooves all hospice professionals to be at least moderately proficient in shame identification and mitigation.

The most important thing for end-of-life professionals to remember when it comes to providing spiritual care is this: If through relationships, shame came into our emotional process, then, through relationships shame can be mitigated, and even transformed. What is needed then from end-of-life professionals is the ability to establish meaningful relationships in the midst of what is likely a shame-saturated environment. There are several qualities of personal and spiritual capacities that end-of-life professionals would do well to develop.

A common aspect of each of these qualities is the realization that spiritual care at the end of life is less about "doing" than it is about "being." This means that it is less important for hospice professionals to "do" therapy or perform therapeutic interventions, than it is for them to be genuine and accepting of that particular family's emotional process. Sometimes this means lingering even when the family seems to want to hurry through the visit. That is, the sense of one's confidence in being in a relationship is more important than many of one's other skills and abilities.

EXPERIENCED SHAME AND ITS TRANSFORMATION

An end-of-life spiritual caregiver should be comfortable with his or her own "woundedness." All of us, to some degree or another, have been "wounded" by shame, and experience our own vulnerability toward being shamed again. An end-of-life spiritual caregiver comes into a family's life at a time when one of their members is dying, and thus enters into a world of people who are highly sensitized to their vulnerability, especially to their shame wounds. Being spiritual caregivers means that we join into caring relationships, and, all the while, we remain aware of our own wounds. In the case of end-of-life spiritual care, we bring our awareness of the wounds of our own chronic shame to bear. This in itself can lead to a profound acceptance of the chronic woundedness from shame that we all carry—individually, and as families.

What makes this a capacity, ability, or skill is that shame is something we reactively turn away from, or even flee. Our learned reaction to the extreme pain of shame was to avoid shame-filled situations and to shun the shamed. We do not easily embrace our own shame, let alone another's or both together.

For end-of-life care professionals to be able to develop relationships with those who are experiencing acute shame, they must be able to move *toward* those in shame, to be willing to reach out to them, and establish a relational contact. In order to be effective in this paradoxical and even contrarian behavior, end-of-life professionals must bring a "healthy" sense of shame to their spiritual care. "Healthy shame is about tact: literally how to be in touch" (Whitehead & Whitehead, 1995, p. 104). We can be in touch with those experiencing shame if we stay in touch with our own. This is the basis of the virtue of humility.

This is why providing spiritual care at the end of life means not only being aware of one's own shame wounds, but also having addressed those wounds sufficiently to have established a healthy sense of shame in oneself. For this is the interaction of spiritual care: The spiritual caregiver is able to hold simultaneously an awareness of his own shame-experience *and* the shame-experience of the patient and/or family—and not absorb the shame of that family's emotional process into his/her own. This is the capacity to *be with* someone at the end of life and to be as aware of *their* shame as one's own—and yet to be comfortable in oneself with that, and with all of that shame. This is how true mutuality is established.

This capacity for *being with* shame develops as one experiences the mitigation and even transformation of one's own shame. From that comes both the confidence that this can happen for and within others, and a sense of self-protection from toxic or malfunctioning shame. That is, when one has experienced having one's own shame mitigated, that very shame becomes like a vaccine against further shame wounding, from additional shame intoxication. The *fear* of being shamed further is released, and in its place comes a comfort with one's own humanity and a confidence to *be with* the humanity of another person.

The irony of this dimension of spiritual care is that it is most likely to have been developed in persons who themselves have experienced AEP. This is because through it, and especially through entering the spiritual process of recovery from it, they are more likely to be shame-sensitive and shame-aware than those who have experienced only FEP.

NONSHAMING PRESENCE

In speaking to capacities for organizational leadership using family systems principles, Edwin Friedman advocated for leadership as "non-anxious presence." His aim was the modification of organizational anxiety. A leader's capacity to be "nonanxious" could do this. He said, "To the extent that we can recognize and contain our own anxiety, then we can function as step-down transformers, or perhaps circuit breakers" (Friedman, 1985, p. 209).

Two aspects of nonanxious presence that Friedman valued were the complementary capacities for being playful, on the one hand, and for avoiding the "dangers of diagnosis" on the other hand. Diagnostic thinking serves to intensify anxiety by heightening the seriousness in the system, and increasing polarization. The antidote for diagnostic thinking Friedman proposed was "playfulness," by which he meant a capacity for paradox and a capacity to relax and remain calm in situations that had become stressed by seriousness (Friedman, 1985, p. 209). Spiritual caregivers at the end of life would be wise to develop both of these aspects of being a nonanxious presence.

Being nondiagnostic and even playful might seem inappropriate at times in life when shame is manifested and palpable. Yet these personal characteristics can be even more beneficial in mitigating and trans-forming shame, perhaps because they also release anxiety.

In fact, sometimes spiritual caregivers learn about the limitations of diagnostic thinking and the benefits of being playful from their patients and families. A classic example is recounted by Mitch Albom (1997) in *Tuesdays with Morrie*. Dying from amyotrophic lateral sclerosis (ALS), Morrie Schwartz had gone public with his fears about when a potentially shaming day would come: He would be incontinent and be unable to clean himself. How Morrie transforms an experience he once feared into one that he finds he enjoys is in itself a story of personal shame mitigation (Albom, 1997, pp. 115–116).

Three aspects of this account are especially worth noting for the shame-transforming virtues that Morrie displays. The first is that, by this time in Morrie's life, it no longer matters what he is dying from. Morrie is no longer an ALS patient, but a person who is dying. His diagnosis has lost almost all meaning; its consequences are simply facts of his everyday life. Morrie's adjustment was what he called "complete surrender to the disease" (p. 115). Such surrender is a sign of Mor-rie's *humility*.

The second is Morrie's capacity to be playful. He has taken a feared eventuality, and chosen to treat it with acceptance—one might even say, a sense of fun. Morrie tells Mitch, "I began to *enjoy* my dependency" (p. 116). He is able to do this because, instead of being embarrassed by his body's regression, he embraces it—he embraces "going back to being a child again" (p. 116). As he tells Mitch:

> The truth is, when our mothers held us, rocked us, stroked our heads— none of us ever got enough of that. We all yearn in some way to return

to those days when we were completely taken care of—unconditional love, unconditional attention. Most of us didn't get enough. I know I didn't. (p. 116)

This in itself is a fine demonstration of having arrived at a healthy sense of shame. Morrie has redefined his *modesty*, to fit what is appropriate for him at that time in his life.

The third aspect is Morrie's attitude toward shame itself. On one hand, Morrie declares his independence from our culture and its expectations. He tells Mitch that, having been an independent person, at first he felt ashamed at all the ways he needed assistance.

I felt ashamed, because our culture tells us we should be ashamed if we can't wipe our own behind. But then I figured, *Forget what the culture says. I have ignored the culture much of my life. I am not going to be ashamed. What's the big deal?* (pp. 115–116)

Here Morrie's independence from cultural influences gives him a certain freedom with respect to his own *dignity*, and choices about how to manage his own shame. In systems' terms, this is a mark of a very well-differentiated person.

On the other hand, Morrie recognizes that his own choice to be independent of cultural constraints might not be the choice of those in whose hands he has placed himself for care. He demonstrates an ability not only to maintain his own dignity but also to preserve the dignity of his caregiver, Connie, when he asks her to clean him after he's used the commode. "Would you be embarrassed to do it for me?" he asks (p. 115). In consulting his caregiver, he demonstrates a concern for *her* shame. In other words, he does not presume that she is as freed from cultural expectations as he is. In establishing his own dignity, he also preserves hers. Morrie's capacity for self-differentiation keeps him aware of and in touch with the feelings of others, exhibiting a healthy sense of belonging.

This is an excellent illustration of a how a healthy sense of shame functions. Worthy of note is that Albom, the observer, does not say that *he* felt ashamed. The moment becomes one of *community*, of coming together, a moment to embrace and to be embraced by.

Spiritual caregivers who develop the capacities to be a presence that is both nonanxious and nonshaming affirm the basic humanity of their patients and their families, beyond the categorization of their diagnosis and the diminution that dying is for many.

Speaking Shame

To take one more aspect from Albom's account, professional spiritual caregivers should note how Morrie *names* the shame, and points to what is embarrassing about dying—the sense of inevitable regression, the felt return to the time in life when shame first became an aspect of psychological development and bodily mastery.

The strength of Morrie's ability to speak of shame is ratified by Brown's (2003) research and shame resilience theory (SRT). One aspect of SRT that can be used in a variety of practice settings entails what in spiritual care would be called "inviting a conversation." In end-of-life care, for example, the spiritual caregiver would, again using Albom's account as an example, make explicit note of Morrie's change in attitude and then, either expressly or tacitly, "invite" Morrie to say still more about how he had done that. Speaking of shame means more than developing a shame vocabulary. It means being willing to *share*, and to create a conversational space wherein talking about shame is comfortable.

Creating this space is a spiritual process, not a psychological or therapeutic one. In fact, participants in Brown's study "rarely identified psychotherapy or individual counseling as an effective tool." Rather, their responses favored: "'being with others who have had similar experiences' or 'talking with people who've been there'" (Brown, 2003, p. 51). In our words, speaking of shame is most effective when there is a felt sense of mutuality.

SUMMARY: LISTENING WITH THE EAR OF THE HEART

An important counterpoint to being able to speak about shame is having the capacity to *listen* to someone else speak their shame. *Listening,* in a spiritual sense, is of course more than merely hearing. It is the capacity to stay *present* in body, mind and spirit. Shame is difficult to voice, but it is also difficult to hear, and those who provide spiritual care could find themselves "abandoning" their patients and their families "in place"—not by physically leaving, but by judging, assessing, categorizing, diverting, deflecting, or otherwise defending themselves from the discomforts that commonly come with shame awareness.

It has been said that "all 'community' begins in *listening*" (Kurtz & Ketcham, 1992, p. 94), and nowhere else is this more true than when providing spiritual care at the end of life. The significance of listening to the mitigation and transformation of shame perhaps can be taken from the Chinese character for shame (*ch'ih*) that juxtaposes the characters for "heart" and "ear" (Whitehead & Whitehead, 1995, p. 90). From it, we take this suggestion: In spiritual care, *when we listen with the ear of the heart, shame is transformed.* There is little or no embarrassment. Instead, when one's heart can hear the shame of another, and one can hold another's shame in one's own heart, then a heartfelt relationship is established—human to human, heart to heart. The consequent experience is a rare and sometimes surprising sense of belonging, a moment of transcendent being together, when we are as present to one another as we are, and yet, unashamed of that vulnerability.

An experience of this kind of belonging is the aim of spiritual care at the end of life. How that goal is reached entails still one other aspect of spiritual care: The importance of stories. What spiritual caregivers should listen *for* are stories. Morrie's account of his making a different choice in how to manage—indeed, *experience*—his shame is misleadingly straightforward in its candor. Most of the time, people tell stories about what this moment means to them, and why. In the narrative structure of their disclosures, patients and families often mean more than they can otherwise say. And sometimes in the telling of it, those meanings in turn become evident to them—and their experience of themselves and of each other is changed, most often for the better. George and Wilma's reminiscing about events in their marriage, for instance, told them that they had loved each other more than just saying those words might have conveyed.

The adept spiritual caregiver invites stories, precisely for the surplus of meaning that is in them. In the course of the story-telling, and the story-listening, often something "more" happens. Perhaps we discover that we are not that different from one another, that in fact, there is this sense that in sharing stories, *all* of our stories are "shared." "Spirituality flourishes in discovery, and especially in the discovery of *shared story*— the discovery that creates community" (Kurtz & Ketcham, 1992, p. 95, emphasis added). In the process, each of our lives is affirmed and a moment of special privilege can be acknowledged, thankfully.

There is transcendence in this experience, a shared sense of the depth and trust of that moment, one that is set apart from the usual and the commonplace. One can tell that this is happening because, in one's own heart, one experiences a sense of gratitude. Along with that gratitude for the moment and everyone in it, flows an experience of that which is greater than oneself.

This, of course, is the ultimate experience of shame transformation any time that it occurs, but especially if it occurs in the waning moments of one's life. The ultimate antidote to addiction, its emotional process, and the shame experienced by any and all of us at one time or another in our lives comes in moments such as these, when shame is transcended by merciful acceptance, and death is transcended by caring love.

REFERENCES

Albom, M. (1997). *Tuesdays with Morrie: An old man, a young man, and life's greatest lesson*. New York: Doubleday.

Bradshaw, J. (1988). *Healing the shame that binds us*. Deerfield Beach, FL: Health Communications.

Brown, B. (2003). Shame resilience theory: A grounded theory study on women and shame. *Families in Society: The Journal of Contemporary Social Services, 87*(1), 43–52.

Dearing, R., Stuewig, J., & Tangney, J. P. (2005). On the importance of distinguishing shame from guilt: Relations to problematic alcohol and drug use. *Addictive Behaviors, 30*(7), 1392–1404.

Erikson, E. H. (1963). *Childhood and society*. New York: W. W. Norton.

Fossum, M. A., & Mason, M. J. (1986). *Facing shame: Families in recovery*. New York: W.W. Norton.

Friedman, E. H. (1985). *Generation to generation: Family process in church and synagogue*. New York: Guilford Press.

Kurtz, E., & Ketcham, K. (1992). *The spirituality of imperfection: Storytelling and the search for meaning*. New York: Bantam Books.

Lee, R. G., & Wheeler, G. (2003). *The voice of shame*. Cambridge, MA: Gestalt Press.

May, G. G. (1988). *Addiction & grace*. San Francisco: Harper.

Morrison, A. P. (2003). Shame: On ideals and idealization. *Annals of the New York Academy of Sciences, 1159*, 75–85.

Scheff, T. J. (2003). Shame in self and society. *Symbolic Interaction, 26*(2), 12–25.

Schneider, C. D. (1992). *Shame, exposure, and privacy*. New York: W. W. Norton.

Wheeler, G. (2003) Shame, guilt and codependency: Dana's world. In R. G. Lee & G. Wheeler (Eds.), *The voice of shame*. Cambridge, MA: Gestalt Press.

Whitehead, J. D., & Whitehead, E. E. (1995). *Shadows of the heart: A spirituality of the negative emotions*. New York: Crossroads.

Afterword: When the Hospice Journey Meets the Road to Recovery: Taking 12 Steps Toward the End of Life*

Now that we have gained an appreciation for how family systems theory can make a positive contribution to end-of-life care, we want to encourage further the possibility for those in recovery from addiction emotional process to enhance the experiences all of us have as we are dying. We would like to suggest the following metaphorical intersection: On the one hand, end-of-life care, in the company of the professionals of the hospice team, could be called the "hospice journey." On the other hand, the aim for health as one recovers from addiction could be called the "road to recovery." Those on the hospice journey and those on the road to recovery may encounter each other precisely at that intersection when persons and families with addiction emotional process come under the care of hospice.

Here we want to explore the ways the 12-Step program's perspective might aid those receiving and providing care at the end of life. Traditionally the 12 Steps have been used to provide spiritual and emotional

---

*Material in this chapter was previously published in DeFord, B., & Bushfield, S. (2008). When the hospice journey meets the road to recovery: Taking 12 steps toward the end of life. *Healing Ministry, 15*(2), 27–34. Reprinted with permission.

guidance to those in recovery from addiction and/or its attendant behaviors. The road to recovery extends toward life: One takes this road in order to live more freely from the binds of addiction, and to improve the quality of one's character and relationships.

The hospice journey heads in a very different direction—toward the close of life, toward death. Yet many in the end-of-life care tradition suggest that "it is not too late," that the process of dying itself can be "the final stage of growth" (Kübler-Ross, 1988), and that given sufficient time and opportunity, one who is dying can make positive changes in himself and in his relationships with others. This way of thinking represents one aspect of "the good death."

Contributing to this tradition, Byock (1997, 2004) sets out what could be called "tasks" for the dying. These four tasks are: To forgive and to ask for forgiveness; to be grateful and to express one's gratitude; to be loving and to express one's love; and to say "good-bye." These tasks provide something to *do*, and serve as a bridge from "doing" to "being," which represents a shift in perspective. For people who are terminally ill, it is empowering to discover that, while there is nothing more that can be done medically, there may still be things for them to do.

In a similar spirit, the 12 Steps offer to those seeking recovery from addiction a path, a series of steps to take or things to do so that they can help themselves. Observing that the 12 Steps are empowering to recovering addicts, we asked ourselves how they might be adapted to be similarly empowering for those at the end of life.

STEP ONE: WE ADMITTED WE WERE POWERLESS OVER OUR ADDICTION—THAT OUR LIVES HAD BECOME UNMANAGEABLE

In Alcoholics Anonymous (A.A.), the First Step toward freedom from alcoholism is the admission about loss of "the power of choice" (Alcoholics Anonymous, 2007, p. 24). This admission is made at a time when significant loss is recognized in other areas of life as well. Thus, the First Step of recovery is taken in a context of what end-of-life care providers might call *grief*. The addict's life has come to grief. The realization that life as it had been lived needs to come to an end is a step *away* from life as the addict knows it. The First Step is made on that cusp between an ending and a beginning.

For the one being given a terminal prognosis, the cusp is similar. Life as it had been lived, with a central purpose of *cure*, is now no longer available. Instead, a new purpose must be found, and a new way of living must be discovered, within a relatively abbreviated horizon of time. In addition, the one who is entering the period of the end of his or her life, does so with a certain powerlessness: One is powerless to make things different; one's life is largely no longer in one's control.

A *First Step* for someone on the hospice journey might be: *I admitted I was powerless to extend my life, powerless over my finite condition—and to that extent, I had to face my loss of control.*

The person at the end of life discovers in the course of dying just to what limited extent one has control and power of choice. In significant respects, this is like the person in recovery: Both experience loss and limitation. Perhaps this is one reason why the Serenity Prayer has become comforting to both populations: *"God, grant me the serenity to accept the things I cannot change; the courage to change the things I can; and the wisdom to know the difference."* For the person traveling the road to recovery or the one taking the hospice journey, this prayer articulates three spiritual gifts one would like to receive: serenity, courage, and wisdom.

In this respect, those on the road to recovery can make those taking the hospice journey more aware of the essentially spiritual quality of their path. Persons at the end of their lives desire serenity, courage and wisdom, and persons on the road to recovery understand that these are hardly personal achievements, but more gifts, granted by God, or as they would say, "the God of one's own understanding" or "Higher Power." It may help people who are at the end of their lives to understand, especially when they are not feeling serene, or courageous, or wise; that serenity, courage and wisdom come to one in quite some other way than by achieving these qualities personally in oneself. In fact, this is what makes *The Serenity Prayer*, a prayer: It is a plea, not a self-affirmation.

To appreciate the importance of spirituality to those on the road to recovery, we need to look at Steps 2 and 3.

STEP TWO: WE CAME TO BELIEVE THAT A POWER GREATER THAN OURSELVES COULD RESTORE US TO SANITY

STEP THREE: WE MADE A DECISION TO TURN OUR WILL AND OUR LIVES OVER TO THE CARE OF GOD AS WE UNDERSTOOD GOD

It is important for A.A. to have participants understand the spiritual nature of the program: "Do not let any prejudice you may have against spiritual terms deter you from honestly asking yourself what they mean to you" (Alcoholics Anonymous, 2007, p. 47). In a similar way, those in hospice often say: "A person may or may not *have* a religion, but everyone *is* spiritual." Thus both the road to recovery and the hospice journey can be thought of as spiritual paths.

Yet there is a difference in their points of view. In hospice, typically, spiritual caregivers would not speak about "God" per se, unless the patient or family member does. Yet in A.A., the term is used with some specificity and purpose. "God" is "a Power greater than myself." The purpose of this understanding is to help the addict get outside or beyond himself. In theological terms, it offers the addict the advantage of a belief in *transcendence*, a belief in something more than the individual's own will and world.

The spirituality of A.A. and other 12-Step Programs is every bit as nonspecific and nonreligious as hospice's. No effort is made to develop a doctrine of God. When A.A. and other 12-Step Programs speak of "God" it is always in this qualified sense: "the God of one's own under-standing." Each person who embarks on the road to recovery is free to discover his own sense of who "God" is and what "God" means to him or her. This is in large part what makes 12-Step Programs spiritual and not religious.

But it is important for participants in 12-Step Programs to have a belief in "God," albeit one of their own understanding, for this reason— humility: The Second Step is essentially a teaching of the benefits of the spiritual quality of humility.[1]

On the road to recovery, the humility of coming to believe in a power greater than oneself leads to faith. With faith comes hope.[2] And with hope comes love and a sense of community.[3] This sense of love and community is reinforced in perhaps the only criterion 12-Step Programs ask their participants to believe about the "God of their own understanding": Namely, that "God" be not only greater than oneself but also loving and caring.[4]

Finally, this "coming to believe" that begins in humility and finds hope, love, and community is all toward a single purpose in 12-Step Programs: the restoration of sanity. This is precisely why the God of one's own understanding *must* be transcendent, or greater than oneself. It replaces the role of the drug of choice. Powerless against using the drug of choice, at the limits of one's own personal capacities, the recovering person places his or her faith in God as being greater than the drug. In doing so, in making the *choice* to believe, the one who would recover and who would be restored puts into place what the *Big Book* calls a "simple cornerstone [for] a wonderfully effective spiritual structure" (A.A., 2007, p. 47).

On the hospice journey, no "spiritual structure" must be built—but one is nonetheless very likely discovered. When one embarks on the hospice journey, one is likely to have experiences that one could find humiliating, provided one does not find a way to face them with humility.[5] Moreover, one struggles with hope; specifically the difference between "hope" itself and "hope for..." and "hope in...." It is to be hoped that one discovers that one is not alone. One certainly discovers something of what love means, and to what extent one has a community of care around oneself. One also may discover whether and to what degree one has already built a "spiritual structure" for oneself. If drug use and abuse and the attendant behaviors could be said to be "death by degrees," then there is something absolute about the *Death* one faces at the end of life. It is this very absolute quality that inspires in people an awareness of their spirituality. We would say that many come to an awareness of the "God of their own understanding" simply by taking the hospice journey.

The 12 Steps encourage one to make that understanding explicit. Thus a *Second Step* for someone on the hospice journey might be: *I came to believe that a Power greater than myself would love and care for me and give me hope as I went toward the end of my life.*

Participants along the road to recovery might encourage those taking the hospice journey to follow the Third Step, thus moving from belief to what we would call *surrender*. The surrendering inherent in the Third Step, in turning over and letting go, for example, benefits those on the road to recovery in specific ways. They speak to the decision to put the faith of the Second Step into action in the Third. What is crucial about the Third Step is this deciding—a sense of taking personal responsibility for one's own life.

This is the marvelously paradoxical spirituality of the 12 Steps. First, there is the confession of personal powerlessness, then the affirmation of faith in a Power greater than oneself. Then there is the encouragement to "at last *abandon* ourselves utterly to Him" (A.A., 2007, p. 63, emphasis added). Through the conscious decision of surrender comes a restoration of the power of choice. This paradox is what makes the 12 Steps a classic spiritual path.

Similarly, for those taking the hospice journey, there is much that needs to be let go of. The spiritual discovery to be made is that the more one is willing to surrender to the parameters of dying, the more one is restored to oneself, the more one finds one's true autonomy and integrity still intact. This paradoxical decision in favor of surrender is essentially what maintains the dignity of the one who is dying.

One could say that a *Third Step* for someone on the hospice journey might be: *I made a decision to turn my life (my past, my present, and my future) over to God, as I understand God to be.*

Whether making the hospice journey or traveling the road to recovery, we are now ready to take the next step.

STEP FOUR: WE MADE A SEARCHING AND FEARLESS MORAL INVENTORY OF OURSELVES

Having taken the first three steps of turning from their addiction and toward the God of their understanding, persons on the road to recovery then take an inward turn, and look at themselves. Of all the steps, many find this one the most challenging, significant, and growth-producing. For it involves being honest—and admitting aspects of oneself that one might otherwise want to deny.

For recovering persons, the moral inventory is a thorough assessment of the character defects and behaviors that have led to their failure and caused them to hurt themselves and others, *and* a listing of their good qualities. To do this, one confronts one's fears and strives for a degree of honesty that might otherwise have been missing. The goal is to "free ourselves of living in old, useless patterns" (Narcotics Anonymous,

2008, p. 28). It is important that this step be taken in a balanced way, so that some aspects of character are retained and emphasized, but other aspects are "modified or discarded" (Nelson, 1990, p. 38).

People who are taking the hospice journey often find themselves in the midst of a similar process. They may not actually choose it, but rather find that it arises for them. Knowing that one is at the end of one's life often prompts this sort of self-assessment or life review. Many, even those not otherwise so inclined, find their minds wandering in this direction at the end of life.

What the Fourth Step can bring to those on the hospice journey is the encouragement that such an assessment can be done *fearlessly*. This is not to be a "pity party," nor a vain effort to prop up false and eroding self-images. Instead the Fourth Step, taken at the end of life, becomes an effort at *authenticity*, a balanced claiming of the ways in which one was good, and did well, versus the ways in which one has failed to live up to the best in oneself, and as a result, has hurt oneself and others.

Thus the *Fourth Step* for someone at the end of life might be: *I made a thorough moral inventory of myself, addressing my fears and my failures, and affirming my essential goodness.*

The Fourth Step may occur repeatedly to those on the road to recovery. But for those on the hospice journey, Fourth Steps might be taken less definitively, more spontaneously, and with less of a sense of opportunity for repetition. Thus a Fourth Step might be as "thorough" as one can be at the time. And it might come with an acceptance that the effort itself was made, however incomplete.

Because of the difference in life circumstance, what one does with what one learns in the Fourth Step might be both different and all the more important for someone taking the hospice journey, for there is a finality to this inventory that adds to its importance at the end of life.

STEP FIVE: WE ADMITTED TO GOD, TO OURSELVES, AND TO ANOTHER HUMAN BEING THE EXACT NATURE OF OUR WRONGS

In taking this next Step, the person on the road to recovery turns outward again. The object of this Step is to overcome a sense of isolation, to work through whatever shame might be masquerading as privacy, to hear oneself "confess" one's own history to another person. This "speaking out loud" has its own salutary effect. As the *Big Book* says, for alcoholics, "they had not learned enough of humility, fearlessness and honesty…, until they told someone *all* of their life story" (A.A., 2007, p. 73).

Again, those taking the hospice journey may essentially discover something similar: A shift occurs in them when they start telling others of their lives and of themselves. These disclosures may seem random to hospice team members, but if we understand the importance of Step 5 to those on the road to recovery, we who provide end-of-life care can better appreciate what might be going on within the emotional processes of the patient and/or family member.

Specifically, it may be important for us in end-of-life care to listen, to receive what we are told, and to respond in a particular way. If we understand persons at the end of life merely to be undergoing what we like to call "life review," then we may miss the moment, and not meet the underlying need. Yet, if we take a page from those in recovery, and seize these times as if those dying were taking a Fifth Step, then we are more likely to respond to what is really being asked of us: A quality of mercy, understanding, and compassion. The need is not only to tell the story, but for someone truly to hear it.

When those in recovery take a Fifth Step, they are risking that another, hearing one's honest and as thorough-going-as-possible self-description, will respond with censure and judgment. Persons in recovery thus choose their listeners carefully, knowing this risk. People who are taking the hospice journey may be making just as careful a choice, but may not have as many others to choose from! Often, for both persons on the road to recovery and those taking the hospice journey, family members and friends are ruled out, because they are already a part of the story being told. It is important for those providing end-of-life care to appreciate, honor, and respect the choice of those on the hospice journey, should they take this Fifth Step. Likewise, family members may need help in understanding, honoring, and respecting the nature of the choice the dying person makes.

For those taking the hospice journey, a *Fifth Step* might be: *I admitted to God, to myself, and to another human being the exact nature of myself and my life, as I understood them to be.*

Those on the hospice journey, like those on the road to recovery, having taken the first Five Steps, find themselves at a different place within themselves, with others perhaps, and most certainly, before God. They are then led to the next two Steps.

STEP SIX: WE WERE ENTIRELY READY TO HAVE GOD REMOVE ALL THESE DEFECTS IN CHARACTER

STEP SEVEN: WE HUMBLY ASKED GOD TO REMOVE OUR SHORTCOMINGS

We have put these two Steps together because the first is preparation for the second. In spiritual terms, the Sixth Step is the moment of stillness that precedes the process of engagement.

For those on the road to recovery, Step 6 is a step of preparation and reflection. It is a pause for consideration before turning oneself over to God once again—this time with the expectation that God *will*, in fact, make a change in oneself and one's life. Making sure one is ready for the change is as important as asking that it be made. For the person on the road to recovery, this pause may allow time to overcome one's resistance or reluctance for God to work in this way before going forward.

In the recovery process, there is an expectation that the change being asked for—and more—will surely come. In recovery literature, the similarity between Steps 3 and 7 is noted: Similar to Step 3, Step 7 is one of surrender, of turning over. The difference is that by Step 7, one's life and self will be changed.

It bears noting that these two steps may be the last that those on the hospice journey are able to take. By the time most people reach this state of mind, by the time they are prepared for a complete surrender to God, they are likely to be quite near death. It is likely that the anticipated transformation eases them from this life into whatever they believe is next. The evidence of God's loving-kindness and mercy will most likely be displayed in how they die. The moment of stillness in preparation for death and the self-conscious submission to death are not necessarily significant moments in the dying process, but occasionally they are articulated by the dying person in preparation for what is to come. For the hospice journey, Steps 6 and 7 would suggest: *I am prepared to die and I am ready for what is to come.*

There is one other quality at the end of life that seems to parallel the road to recovery: *Humility*. The wording of Step 7 says as much, but as one source stated, "taking Step Seven was for many of us the greatest act of authentic humility we have ever been asked to commit: to transfer control of our recovery to God...." (Miller, 2007, p. 116).

By the same token, most of us come to the end of our lives quite humbled by the dying process. Whether we find an acceptance of that, and thus realize a humility we may never before have experienced, or still resist and feel humiliated by it, very much determines what our experience of dying will be—and how others experience our dying. If humility is the open ground for the God of our understanding to bring about profound change in us, then it is the common goal for both those on the road to recovery and those taking the hospice journey.

STEP EIGHT: WE MADE A LIST OF ALL PERSONS WE HAD HARMED, AND BECAME WILLING TO MAKE AMENDS TO THEM ALL

STEP NINE: WE MADE DIRECT AMENDS TO SUCH PEOPLE WHEREVER POSSIBLE, EXCEPT WHEN TO DO SO WOULD INJURE THEM OR OTHERS

For those on the road to recovery, taking each of these steps one at a time is an essential aspect of spiritual growth. They have already opened themselves to God, and surrendered to God's transformation. Now they are turning to other people. Recovery is not only about what occurs *within*; it is also about what occurs *between*: between themselves and God, and between themselves and others.

Just as Step 6 was preparation for Step 7, Step 8 is one of preparation for Step 9. Step 8 is sometimes called a "social housecleaning" just as Step 4 was a "personal housecleaning" (Miller, 2007, p. 135). It entails the significant recognition that living in this world is all about *relationships*, and that having lived as one did, those relationships were damaged—one did harm.

If Step 8 is about the preparation to make amends, then Step 9 is the carrying through of the action. A genuine consideration of the other comes into play, for with Step 9 comes the assessment of how the other would feel about or otherwise be affected by one's effort to make amends. For in both steps, the amends-making is being done *for oneself*, for one's own benefit, but it is also very important to ask, perhaps for the first time, how others will feel, what they will think, and how they will be affected by this reaching out to make amends for one's past behavior.

This is no small consideration on the part of the recovering addict, especially since this discernment is to be made on the basis of an assessment of where the other is now, *not* on the basis of one's own willingness to carry through with the amends. As the *Big Book* says, "we may lose our position or reputation or face jail, but we are willing. We have to be. We must not shrink at anything" (A.A., 2007, p. 79).

Because it entails giving consideration to the life situation of others, these Steps may take some time for those on the road to recovery, especially if they are to be accomplished thoroughly. That is why, when it comes to Steps 8 and 9, the model provided by the road to recovery might exceed the capacity of most persons taking the hospice journey. There simply may be limitations of time and of consciousness.

This is not to say that forgiveness, which is one aspect of the process, is not important to those coming to the end of their lives. Byock (2004), among others, has discussed how the giving of, asking for, and (hopefully) receiving of forgiveness can be a pivotal part of one's spiritual life as one approaches death.

Certainly the road to recovery can be helpful to those on the hospice journey in this respect: Quite often people seem to come to the brink of death, and linger. When this happens, it is likely that family, friends, and often even hospice caregivers will frame this as the person's not "letting go" of life, but rather of their "holding on"—for some reason. While that reason may never be known, we speculate whether the dying person is not waiting to hear a word of forgiveness.

Often, the dying person hears words of "permission"—"It's OK. You can go now." Sometimes those words seem efficacious, which is to say, the person dies after they are spoken. However, we wonder whether the dying person is not wanting to hear something else; perhaps: "I hope you will forgive me"; or "I want you to know that I've forgiven you." When framed in a context of forgiveness, this one-sided dialogue, to which the dying person makes scant if any response, can be more emotionally and spiritually satisfying for the survivor. This is because the context of forgiveness is one of mutuality, while the context of permission is one of "control"—over a process neither the survivor nor the one dying truly has any power. In a word, the context of forgiveness is more authentic than the context of permission. Forgiveness might also be viewed as an empowering gift—not given to only another, but a gift given primarily to one's self, as acknowledgment that what is forgiven no longer wields power and control. In this context, we move from forgiveness (for that for which one was guilty and needed atonement) to acceptance (for that which was held to be shameful). The person in recovery learns that it is possible to take responsibility for one's self and one's actions, whether or not others respond. Perhaps at the end of life, the one dying can also take steps toward forgiveness and acceptance, whether or not others respond. For that reason, Steps 8 and 9 for those on the hospice journey might be: *I am ready to forgive and be forgiven.*

There is one other key difference between those in recovery and those at end of life. To the degree that making amends involves more than just forgiveness but also perhaps restitution, those on the hospice journey may be significantly less able to take such actions than those on the road to recovery. Still, occasionally those on the hospice journey do want to "make things right" before they die. And those on the road to recovery have a deep understanding of why this might be important.

STEP TEN: WE CONTINUED TO TAKE PERSONAL INVENTORY AND WHEN WE WERE WRONG PROMPTLY ADMITTED IT

STEP ELEVEN: WE SOUGHT THROUGH PRAYER AND MEDITATION TO IMPROVE OUR CONSCIOUS CONTACT WITH GOD AS WE UNDERSTOOD GOD, PRAYING ONLY FOR KNOWLEDGE OF GOD'S WILL FOR US AND THE POWER TO CARRY THAT OUT

STEP TWELVE: HAVING HAD A SPIRITUAL AWAKENING AS THE RESULT OF THESE STEPS, WE TRIED TO CARRY THIS MESSAGE TO OTHER ADDICTS, AND TO PRACTICE THESE PRINCIPLES IN ALL OUR AFFAIRS

On the road to recovery, we come to the three steps meant to continue to show us the path. In some ways, for those on the road to recovery, the Steps circle back on each other. Throughout recovery one may need to begin again, or to repeat an earlier Step or series of Steps in order to make progress in one's spiritual growth throughout life.

Although he road to recovery is about living, the hospice journey is about dying; whereas the road to recovery is about making new beginnings, the hospice journey is about making respectful, authentic endings.

For this reason, Steps 10, 11, and 12 might seem to be less instructive or encouraging for those on the hospice journey. Even in 12-Step literature there is the sense that these last three steps are about "maintenance" or continued and expanded practice. Step 12, in particular, encapsulates a need to do service—to reach out to other addicts and make known the benefits of the Program.

In spite of how they initially appear, when Steps 10, 11, and 12 are analogously applied to those taking the hospice journey, given factors of time and awareness, they could be taken as emphasizing the *transformative quality* of what we have come to call "a good death." That is, one's dying process transforms the entire family, as the family system renegotiates roles and relationships. For caregivers, the realization may come painfully that their lives are forever changed by their loved one's dying. This new understanding often results in a commitment to helping others in creating and supporting a community of care. For many, this shift in perspective marks a turning point in their mourning, and may lead to an altruistic "giving back" in an effort to incorporate new meaning into a changed life.

The good death can become itself an act of service. How we die leaves a lasting impression on those who survive. We can see the evidence of this in the fact that so many who were served by hospice come to volunteer in hospice, in order to give something back.

This in turn means to us that both the road to recovery and the hospice journey are about *transformation*: About how positive changes come to our lives; and about how the desire awakens in us to offer others a like opportunity. For those providing care along the hospice journey, the loss of a loved one can lead to a discovery of a sense of purpose, often in the name of the one who has died.

Certainly the road to recovery is more than the sum of its 12 Steps. The road to recovery, we have said, is itself a *spiritual* path. As the *Big Book* says: "We have entered the world of the Spirit. Our next function is to grow in understanding and effectiveness" (A.A., 2007, p. 84). Other 12-Step writings make this same affirmation. For example, in *A*

Hunger for Healing, Miller (2007) writes that because "Step 11 provides daily spiritual maintenance," the practice of daily meditation and prayer is pursued. People in recovery pray daily, he writes, "because they feel gratitude, love and a sense of awe that the One with whom they are in contact is using his power to heal them" (Miller, 2007, p. 180). No wonder that Step 12 affirms the "spiritual awakening" of those on the road to recovery. Others are invited to travel that road precisely because of the *joy* it brings, the restoration of *joie de vivre* in the traveler.

We who companion those on the hospice journey know (sometimes more than those who are on it themselves) that time is indefinite: Sometimes the journey is short, but quite often it takes longer than might have been first imagined. Why not then take from the experience of those on the road to recovery that the hospice journey is itself about "spiritual awakening?" Along the way, one might indeed be surprised by a restoration of *joie de vivre,* particularly as one attends to spiritual matters during this time of life. In so living one's last chapter, one can provide an example for others, both in the facing of death, and in the going forth through grief into life. Are not these attitudes essentially what Steps 10, 11, and 12 are about?

We believe that when people embark on the hospice journey, they have indeed, in the words of the *Big Book,* "entered the world of the Spirit" (A.A., 2007, p. 89). We also find in the 12 Steps a basic guide or map for them, one that can bring "spiritual awakening" to them, just as it does for those traveling the road to recovery.

A FINAL WORD: IT'S ALL ABOUT HEALING

In conclusion, we believe that the 12 Steps might provide a framework for understanding what one is experiencing at the end of life, an understanding that could be uniquely beneficial for all of those involved.

For those providing end-of-life care, a 12-Step approach could serve as a significant alternative to what is commonly the present model, namely the so-called "stages" of dying first articulated by Kübler-Ross (1969). Although ground-breaking at the time, "stage" language has proved problematic. In fact, as we noted earlier in this text, Kübler-Ross's five stages have become so qualified as to be repudiated by knowledgeable clinicians. Even though Kübler-Ross herself came to have difficulty with the term "stages," her own misgivings have not prevented the original conception from staying in the popular mind.

There are two ways in which Kübler-Ross's original terminology has been misleading. First, the sequencing that the "stage" language conceptualizes gives clinicians pause and often fails to match the experience of those who are actually approaching the end of their lives. The five stages Kübler-Ross named are more accurately *emotions*—and emotions are seldom experienced in a neat sequence. Moreover, the last stage—acceptance—never did seem to be an adequately descriptive term. Terms such as "resolution" or "resolve" have been suggested and used by many professionals, but even they have been judged to be only fairly accurate.

The 12-Step framework, with its sense of progression and progress, with its presentation of tasks to be done as one is able, and with its general descriptions to be *lived* by those who choose it, would seem to provides a model that is less based on emotion and be more practical and adaptable. That is, instead of describing the emotional progress of those at the end of life, hospice professionals could speak of which "step" such individuals are taking, and their personal progress along the hospice journey thus be duly recognized.

Another benefit of the 12 Steps is that they would provide an understanding of "healing" and what that might mean for those on the hospice journey. On the one hand, for persons at the end of their lives, when they were patients, they sought healing and they thought of healing as being cured of what ailed them. Once they left behind their patient-status and returned to personhood, albeit now as persons at the end of life, they are likely still to be seeking "healing" of some sort. However, they are likely to be at a loss for how to think of that healing that does not include the absence of their disease. The 12-Step model would give them a framework and a language within which to speak about healing in their lives, and in their relationships, but not necessarily the healing of their bodies. How they might *feel* about the way that they are dying might still be expressed in any of the terms that Kübler-Ross identified—and others as well. But their understandings of what they are facing and how to face it, their language for articulating the importance of this particular time in their life to them, could sharpen were they to become familiar with a 12-Step approach.

Finally, for caregivers and companions of those who are dying, a 12-Step model provides a unique framework for understanding their role and shaping their expectations. That is, within the 12-Step framework, they, too, might grow; they, too, might take advantage of this significant time in their lives, as they transition from being caregivers and companions of the dying, into a time of loss and the life-adjustments consequent to grief. We have observed that it is not only persons who are dying that seek healing, but also those who are caring for them, their family and their friends. With a 12-Step framework in place, all of those taking the hospice journey have an opportunity for healing along the way.

NOTES

1. As one text puts it: "Whether agnostic, atheist, or former believer, we can stand together on this Step. True humility and an open mind can lead us to faith…" (A.A., 1981, p. 33).
2. "In spite of all of the failures in my own life—all of the broken promises, hard feelings, disappointments, failures, destructive behavior, hatred, anxiety, depression or guilt in my life—there is still hope. There is hope because there is a Power greater than myself" (retrieved from http://12Step.org).
3. "This person is not alone; there are other caring brothers and sisters who really do understand.…" (Miller, 2007, p. 35).
4. "Our understanding of a Higher Power is up to us. No one is going to decide for us. We can call it the group, the program, or we can call it God. The only suggested guidelines are that this Power be loving, caring and greater than ourselves" (Narcotics Anonymous, 2008, p. 24).
5. Perhaps the most familiar example of this is Morrie Schwartz's experiences with incontinence in Mitch Albom's book, *Tuesdays with Morrie* (1997).

REFERENCES

Abom, M. (1997). *Tuesdays with Morrie*. New York: Random House.

Alcoholics Anonymous. (1981). *Twelve steps and twelve traditions*. New York: A.A. World Services.

Alcoholics Anonymous. (2007). *The big book online* (4th ed.). New York: A.A. World Services. Retrieved April 30, 2008, from http://www.aa.org/bigbookonline

Bill W. (1957). *Alcoholics Anonymous comes of age*. New York: A.A. Publishing.

Byock, I. (1997). *Dying well*. New York: Riverhead Books.

Byock, I. (2004). *The four things that matter most*. New York: Free Press.

Kübler-Ross, E. (1969). *On death and dying*. New York: Scribner.

Kübler-Ross, E. (1988). Death: The final stage of growth. In S. Groff & M. Livingston-Valier (Eds.), *Human survival and consciousness evolution* (pp. 274–285). Albany, NY: University of New York Press.

Miller, J. K. (2007). *A hunger for healing.* New York: HarperCollins.

Narcotics Anonymous. (2008). *Basic text* (6th ed.). Van Nuys, CA: World Service Office.

Nelson, T. (1990). *Serenity: A companion for 12 step recovery.* Nashville, TN: Thomas Nelson Publishing.

Index

CPSIA information can be obtained at www.ICGtesting.com
Printed in the USA
BVOW06s1203090915

417156BV00009B/47/P